⋘⋞⋟⋙

Michael Mosesson's offerings in *Fibrinogen Memoirs 3* chronicles noteworthy events and experiences from his life and research career. The narratives highlight former colleagues and teachers, scientists and academicians, family members, notably his wife, Shirley, close or personal associations, including his friends. (I am honored to be in the last category). They reveal previously unexamined aspects of the life and achievements of a 'Renaissance Man' who has earned that title for his many accomplishments and eclectic lifestyle. The rich and textured fabric of these stories should be used not to judge him, but rather to understand him.

~ *Seth R. Banks*

Other books by Michael Mosesson

FIBRINOGEN MEMOIRS: Journeys of a Clot Doctor
Michael W. Mosesson
IPBooks © 2020

FIBRINOGEN MEMOIRS 2:
The Rise and Fall of the Fibrin Cross-linking Controversy
Michael W. Mosesson
IPBooks © 2022

FIBRINOGEN
W. Nieuwenhuizen, M.W. Mosesson, M de Matt, eds.
Annals of The New York Academy of Sciences. Vol 936:1-643, 2001

MOLECULAR BIOLOGY OF FIBRINOGEN AND FIBRIN
M.W. Mosesson and R.F. Doolittle, eds.
Annals of The New York Academy of Sciences. Vol 408:1-672, 1983

FIBRINOGEN MEMOIRS 3

Ripples on the Water

FIBRINOGEN MEMOIRS 3

Ripples on the Water

Michael W. Mosesson

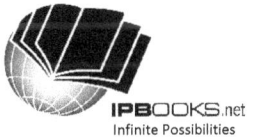

IPBOOKS.net
Infinite Possibilities

Fibrinogen Memoirs 3: Ripples on the Water
By Michael W. Mosesson

Published by IPBooks, Queens, NY
www.IPBooks.net

ISBN 978-1-956864-55-7

Cover concept: Michael W. Mosesson
Front & back cover design: Kathy Kovacic
Editing, typesetting & interior formatting: lisa roma
All photography copyright Michael W. Mosesson,
except where otherwise cited

DEDICATION

This one is for you, Shirley.

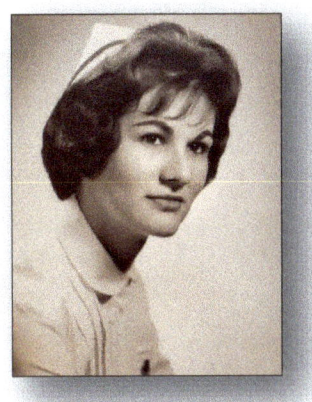

TABLE OF CONTENTS   PAGE

PREFACE

This is the final volume of *Fibrinogen Memoirs*. I chose that title because each story or experience provided is linked, directly or indirectly, to my career in fibrinogen research. I dedicated the first volume to *John Ferry*, a renowned polymer chemist, scientist, educator, linguist, and friend who provided bedrock information on fibrin clot assembly more than seventy years ago. Ferry postulated that fibrin molecules self-assemble in a staggered overlapping manner to form double-stranded fibrils that further associate laterally to form thick fibers displaying a periodicity of 22.5 nm that corresponds to one-half the length of a 45 nm fibrin molecule. To underscore the importance of that construct, I placed an electron micrographic image of a fibrin clot network on the cover page whose fibers showed the expected 22.5 nm spacing.

In the first book I described my upbringing and education in Brooklyn, New York, and the events that led to my career in hemostasis and fibrinogen research. I included a story on aspects of my flying career that began at the time I first began to study fibrinogen. In other sections I described many of the fibrinogen and fibrinogen-related projects and discoveries in which I was involved, with particular attention to a Ferry-inspired chapter entitled *Fibrin, The Perfect Bioelastomer*, in which I proposed that there was an ineluctable relationship between fibrin elasticity and *transverse* positioning of cross-linked gamma chain bonds.

There is also a chapter on the origins and founding of The International Fibrinogen Research Society (IFRS). The narrative is anchored by a chapter written by my friend and colleague, *John Finlayson*, describing the times we spent together at The Laboratory of Blood and Blood Products (LBBP), and the eventual transition of LBBP to become a subsidiary of the Food and Drug Administration (FDA).

Fibrinogen Memoirs 2 is devoted in its entirety to the extant controversy on fibrin cross-linking. It contains bio-sketches and caricatures of scientists who were involved in the discourse, detailed descriptions and interpretive analyses of contributing experimental elements, plus a robust exposition of the structural requirements that accounted for the nearly perfect elasticity of fibrin clots.

In *Fibrinogen Memoirs 3*, I chronicled previously untold events and experiences, all of which were linked to my career as a physician/scientist. They include a story about *Raymond Damadian*, a wannabe Nobel laureate, a detailed description of *The Milwaukee Heart Project* that resulted in the development of a total artificial heart device (TAH), and a tale about a flawed investigator whose unprecedented antics undermined and disrupted the peer review process.

In another chapter, I described the events that contributed to the demise of the cross-linking controversy, one of them at its zenith and the other during its sunset. I also write about *Jim Maroney*, an aviation legend, and in another chapter, I describe my role in CPR on a golf course. Also included is an account of my courtship and marriage to *Shirley Ann McDowell*, including the path to my recovery from grief after her death. That section was followed by a story explaining the provenance of my spiritual fantasy about my grandson, *Sebastian Eckmann*. The final chapter, *Life with The Temkin Tribe*, concerns my long and ultimately convoluted relationship with *Libby Temkin*.

The trilogy provides a description of pathways I pursued in becoming a physician/scientist, summaries of my accomplishments and discoveries, with particular attention to the history and analytical dissection of the fibrin cross-linking controversy. I also describe many professional and personal encounters and experiences. I hope that collectively, they will contribute to my legacy as a scientist, pilot, friend, adversary, father, husband, historian, and storyteller.

Michael Mosesson

Chapter 1
A LIFE CHANGING EVENT IN BOSTON

Medical school at SUNY Downstate was a safe and happy harbor for me. I easily absorbed all the biological, biochemical, and pharmacological course matter and was adept at linking that information with clinical topics and human disease. I had always intended to merge my career as a physician with basic and clinical research. I also believed that achieving that goal would be easier if I could garner a medical residency on an 'elite' service such as the Harvard Medical Service at Boston City Hospital (BCH).

During my second year at SUNY Downstate I spent a research-oriented elective clerkship with *Professor Victor Schenker*, a biochemist in the Psychiatry Department. Schenker wanted to isolate and characterize a bioactive amine secreted by salivary glands. He named the activity *Spitnik,* a name inspired by the satellite, *Sputnik,* that had recently been placed into orbit by The Soviet Union.

Schenker asked me to develop a bioassay for Spitnik using rabbit aortic strips to detect and measure the activity. After I had succeeded in that effort, he used the assay to detect and quantify activity in isolates from human salivary glands. That achievement heightened my interest in an academic research career.

The following year, I became interested in the cardio-pulmonary bypass device (the 'bubble oxygenator') being developed by the chairman of Surgery, *Clarence Dennis*, and I spent another clerkship working in his laboratory on that project. Dennis must have been impressed with my performance because when I broached the subject of a potential surgical career on his service, he enthusiastically suggested that I first spend two years as a house officer on a medical service before beginning a surgical residency in his department at Kings County Municipal Hospital in Brooklyn. When I showed interest in that career path, he offered to support my candidacy for medical residency.

I also spent time with *Professor William Dock* (nicknamed 'Doctor Dock'}, a world-renowned cardiologist/internist who had invented the 'ballistocardiograph', a platform device that could measure headward and footward oscillations produced by the beating heart of a subject who had been positioned on the platform. Dock hoped that ballistocardiography would become a useful clinical tool for investigating cardiac valvular and myocardial abnormalities, but the device was unattractive for commercial development and was never marketed.

The time and effort I spent with Doctor Dock learning the intricacies of his invention must have impressed him because he joined Clarence Dennis in promoting my candidacy for medical residency. With those two icons in my corner, I obtained a position on the II & IV Medical Services (Harvard Service) at BCH.[1] I was the first SUNY-Downstate graduate to obtain such a prestigious appointment. I was on course!

During my first few weeks on the Harvard unit, there were two disturbing incidents that raised doubts in my mind as to whether I was in the right place. One of them occurred when my senior resident for that day, *Harry Jacob*, explained to me how determined he was to minimize patient admissions on his watch.

A short time later he approached a new patient who had just arrived on our floor complaining of anterior chest pain (i.e., a suspected MI!). Jacob motioned for me to accompany him as he

---

[1] At that time, Boston City Hospital had three separate medical services. They were affiliated with three Boston medical schools: Tufts University, Boston University, and Harvard University. The Harvard Service (the II & IV) was reputed to be on the same elite level as the one at Massachusetts General Hospital.

approached the patient holding a colonoscope. While brandishing the scope, he told the cowering patient that he intended to perform a colonoscopy (a procedure that is contra-indicated in subjects with chest pain of unknown etiology). Jacob was hoping that the patient would refuse the procedure and then voluntarily discharge himself by signing out AMA ('Against Medical Advice'). I was appalled at this inappropriate and unethical behavior, and I told him so. In the end, Harry did not follow through with his threat, but the emotional damage to the patient could not be undone.

A few days later, there was another disturbing event. *Thomas Merigan*, the senior resident on duty that evening, abandoned me while I was attempting to stabilize a patient with delirium tremens (DTs), cirrhosis of the liver, and upper GI bleeding, presumably due to bleeding esophageal varices[2]. The patient urgently needed placement of a balloon catheter (a *Sengstaken-Blakemore* tube) to mitigate, if possible, the loss of blood. Merigan appeared in the doorway with several medical journals tucked under his armpit, just after I had inserted the Sengstaken tube into the patient's stomach. I asked Tom to help me inflate the catheter balloon and position it at the esophageal/gastric junction under proper tension.

Merigan looked at me and commented, *"You're doing good guy. Don't forget to do a platelet count when you have time and let me know what the count is. I'll be in the library."*

He then departed, leaving me alone to deal with an agitated patient in a life-threatening situation. Although it was difficult to accomplish by myself, I was finally able to position the catheter

---

[2] Boston City Hospital was known as Mayor *James Curley's* 'home' for the homeless, alcoholics, and other down-and-outers. He was renowned for befriending Boston street people. When these folks turned up at the BCH emergency room looking for a place to stay, whether sick or not, they reportedly said *"Mayor Curley sent me!"* That ploy usually worked, even when the mayor no longer held office.

properly and temporarily stabilize the bleeding, but the eventual outcome for the patient was grim.

After about five weeks at BCH, I received an invitation to meet with *Charles Davidson,* the director of the clinical service, to discuss my experiences to date. Davidson was an outwardly cheerful man who frequently bellowed *'Ho! Ho! Ho!'* whenever given the opportunity. During our meeting he asked me whether I planned to spend a second year on their service. Because of the unsavory incidents described above, that choice had become an issue for me.

I responded, *"I'd like to delay answering your question for a few days. I'll let you know in a week."*

Davidson nodded his acceptance and the meeting ended with another hearty 'Ho! Ho! Ho!'

After thinking about my situation for the next few days, I realized that I had few viable options, and I decided to stay at BCH for a second year. Three days later I went to Davidson's office to convey that decision.

After entering his office, I said deferentially, *"Dr. Davidson, I would like to stay for another year."*

I was surprised when he responded that the position was no longer available. It had been awarded to *Sandor Shapiro,* a former BCH intern who would be returning to replace me. I exited Davidson's office in shock.

It was clear that Charlie Davidson had been looking for an opportunity to bring Shapiro back to BCH. My brief hesitance in making a decision had provided that opportunity. During the next few days, I mulled things over. Should I contact Professor Dennis and ask to begin my surgical residency a year sooner than anticipated? Should I enlist in the Air Force or the Army to advance my clinical training and satisfy the existing government requirement for service in the uniformed services? Should I take a year off to think things over, or perhaps earn some money by freelancing for a year as *locum tenens*? None of the options was appealing.

The Event

A few days after the interview with Davidson, I received an invitation to meet with *William B. Castle*, the Chairman of the Harvard Medical Service at BCH. Among his many achievements and awards, he was a member of The National Academy of Sciences, and he held the George Minot[3] Professor of Medicine Chair at Harvard Medical School. I was awed at the prospect of meeting him.

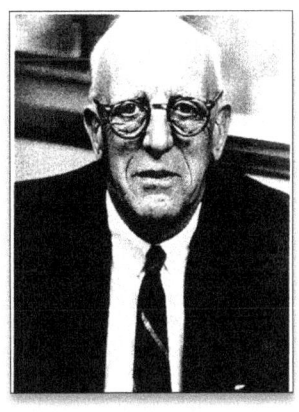

Castle's most well-known scientific/clinical contribution came from his investigations into the pathophysiology of an often-fatal blood disorder, *pernicious anemia*. He and his colleagues at The Thorndike Memorial Laboratory at BCH identified a substance produced by gastric parietal cells (*'gastric intrinsic factor'*) that was necessary for absorption of Vitamin B_{12} (*'extrinsic factor'*), the vitamin that was deficient in pernicious anemia subjects with a stomach secretory disorder called *achylia gastrica*. Vitamin B_{12} in liver accounted for Minot's[3] success in mitigating anemia in their patients.

Castle's work revealed the causal relationship between the anemia in subjects with achylia gastrica and their failure to secrete 'intrinsic factor', aka *'Castle's Factor'*. That discovery, in addition to other clinical research accomplishments, had elevated him to

---

[3] George R. Minot, George H. Whipple, and William P. Murphy shared the 1934 Nobel Prize in Physiology or Medicine for their "discoveries concerning liver therapy in cases of anemia".

legendary status in the medical world.

I had heard Castle speak at our medical conferences and on clinical rounds, but I had not spoken with him directly. That was about to change as I entered his office. He put me at ease immediately by initiating a conversation about my experiences on his service. I did not mention the recent disturbing incidents, but instead extolled features of being a house officer on his service. After a few minutes, he changed the subject to my upcoming unemployment. He remarked that it was unfortunate that I would not be staying at BCH for a second year, and he assured me that I'd be welcomed back at a later date to continue medical training if I so chose.

He then told me about *Sandor (Sandy) Shapiro*, the physician who would be replacing me. Sandy had previously spent one year as an intern at BCH before transferring to The Division of Biologic Standards (DBS) in Bethesda, Maryland in The Laboratory of Blood and Blood Products (LBBP)[4]. With the same stroke he enlisted in the PHS and was stationed at DBS *in lieu* of military service. After spending three years at DBS, he would be returning to BCH to resume residency training.

Castle had been instrumental in brokering both ends of Shapiro's deal, and he was now suggesting that he could arrange the same deal for me. I considered that possibility for only a day or two. The more I thought about it, the more interesting it seemed to be. It was not long before I accepted Castle's offer.

The Course Correction

On July 1, 1960, there was a 'changing of the guard', as aptly phrased by my former colleague, *John Finlayson*, and I arrived at

---

[4] Many of the laboratory and regulatory components of DBS (e.g., virology, LBBP) were subsequently absorbed into The US Food and Drug Administration (FDA).

LBBP in Bethesda. Sandy and I had crossed non-intersecting paths enroute to our new positions, his at BCH and mine at LBBP. We did not meet in person until several years later when he had become Chief of Hematology at The Cardeza Foundation at Thomas Jefferson University in Philadelphia, and I had relocated from Washington University in St. Louis to New York for an academic appointment at SUNY-Downstate Medical Center. It did not take very long before we developed a close and enduring friendship that lasted until his death in 2003 (see Volume 1 of Fibrinogen Memoirs).

Being located at LBBP assured that I would be exposed to the regulatory and research environment of an agency that was responsible for blood bank licensure and oversight, certification or licensing of blood and blood products, fibrinolytic agents, antibodies, vaccines, and other biologicals. Among my regulatory duties I became a blood bank inspector, and in that capacity, I spent considerable time investigating fraudulent updating of donated blood units at several blood banks.

My first laboratory research assignment was to develop an assay for identifying and quantifying the components of commercial fibrinolytic agents then under consideration for licensure. That project required me to learn about *blood coagulation* and *fibrinolysis* in general, and *fibrinogen* and *fibrin* in particular. Within four months I had figured out how to prepare *plasminogen-free fibrinogen*, a critical component for that assay, and a few weeks later I had worked out assay conditions for measuring the components in fibrinolytic products. That achievement eventually led to their licensure and perhaps more importantly, my change in direction.

My first peer-reviewed scientific publication was entitled *Preparation and Properties of Human Fibrinogen Free of Plasminogen* (Biochim Biophys Acta 57, 204-13, 1962) (see Chapter 3 of Fibrinogen Memoirs, volume 1). The experiments that were involved in its production led to other inquiries that yielded

7

considerable data 'fallout' that raised new issues and new inquiries. I was able to address several of them before I left LBBP, but many extended well beyond that period, some lasting until my research career had ended.

By the end of my tour in The Public Health Service I was hooked on blood coagulation, fibrinogen, fibrin, and fibrinolysis. That addiction became the focus of my investigative activities for the next fifty-five years. Alternative career choices that I had once considered, faded from view and never returned. The life changing 'course correction' that resulted from the meeting with *William Castle* led to numerous other lifestyle changes that included marriage to Shirley Ann McDowell, our children, new friends, colleagues and associates, my linguistic pursuits, and more leisurely activities that included a fifty-year flying career. I have disclosed many of them in these volumes of *Fibrinogen Memoirs*.

Michael Mosesson

Chapter 2

RAYMOND DAMADIAN'S QUEST FOR A NOBEL PRIZE

Raymond Vahan Damadian was born to Armenian- American parents and raised in Forest Hills, Queens, New York. In his youth he was a member of the Forest Hills Tennis Club, an organization that hosted the annual US Open Tennis Tournament. Raymond excelled at tennis and squash [as I learned from personal experience while we were faculty members at The SUNY Downstate Medical Center (SUNY-DMC)] and he also studied violin at Juilliard School of Music. He earned an MD degree at Albert Einstein College of Medicine and then became a Ford Foundation Scholar at The University of Wisconsin in Madison, where he developed an interest in Biophysics that led him to the discoveries he made in the field of Nuclear Magnetic Resonance (NMR).

I met Damadian shortly after I had relocated from Washington University in St Louis to join the faculty in The Department of Medicine at SUNY-DMC in Brooklyn in 1967. Like me, he had been recruited by *Ludwig Eichna*, the Chairman of the Department of Internal Medicine. From the outset of his tenure at SUNY-DMC Damadian showed little interest in clinical work, and Eichna for his part, made few such demands on his faculty. That attitude reflected Eichna's recognition of the diversity among his faculty and allowed Raymond to focus almost entirely on investigating Nuclear Magnetic Resonance (NMR) and related subject matter.

NMR is now more popularly termed Magnetic Resonance Imaging (MRI) and has been exploited as an imaging technique featuring significant advantages over standard radiological imaging techniques, including the higher image resolution and the capability to distinguish normal from cancerous tissues based upon the NMR signal from water molecules.

Our research laboratories and offices were in the same wing of the clinical center, and since we both were intensely involved in research, albeit different subject areas, we developed a close friendship. As one aspect of that friendship, we often played squash against each other. These encounters made me realize what an intense and persistent competitor Raymond was. In addition, we had many enlightening and animated discussions, typically during lunch when we talked about our scientific interests and endeavors. It was in that setting that I learned about his ideas concerning NMR as an imaging technique and its potential as a diagnostic/therapeutic modality for diseases such as cancer.

Raymond had a unique way of showing his respect for my scientific achievements. One day during lunch he casually remarked, "Mosesson, you are a two incher!"

"What is that?" I asked, surreptitiously grabbing at my crotch.

It was his version of a compliment. The explanation for that statement is quite simple: There was a weekly publication called *Science Citation Index* that reported the most recent cover or index pages of most biological/biophysical/biochemical periodicals. It also listed the number of times a given author's publications had been cited by others. Damadian would measure the length in inches of any given author's list. He decided that any author whose citation list was longer than one inch was worthy of mention.

In that context, my two inches worth of science citations warranted his respect. As one might have imagined, his own author citation list far exceeded two inches in length, and he was extremely proud of that!

Our lunch discussions also focused on the mechanism of transport of sodium ions (Na+) across cell membranes.[5] The issue of concern was the mechanism by which Na+ ions were transported from the inside to the outside of a cell take place. The prevailing notion, then as now, was that Na transport involved an energy-dependent process catalyzed by an enzyme called Sodium ATPase, although that specific enzyme had yet to be definitively identified and isolated.

Damadian had a unique idea about cellular sodium transport. He had calculated that it was an 'energy catastrophe' insofar as the energy that would be required to drive such a process enzymatically. Instead, he concluded that sodium ion transport to the outside of a cell took place by 'ion exchange'.[6] There was no firm evidence to support his or any other hypothesis at that time.

I was not aware that Raymond's ion exchange hypothesis had been strongly influenced by his belief that *Intelligent Design* accounted for biological processes such as evolution and organs such as eyes. Years after we both had departed from SUNY-DMC, I learned that he became a 'born-again-Christian' at a *Billy Graham* crusade in 1957. Since that conversion he also became an advocate for *Intelligent Design,* an advocacy that included stints on the Advisory Board of the *Institute for Creation Science.*[7]

I am unable to reconcile Damadian's prodigious scientific productivity and creativity with his unfailing allegiance to *Intelligent Design* concepts of evolution.

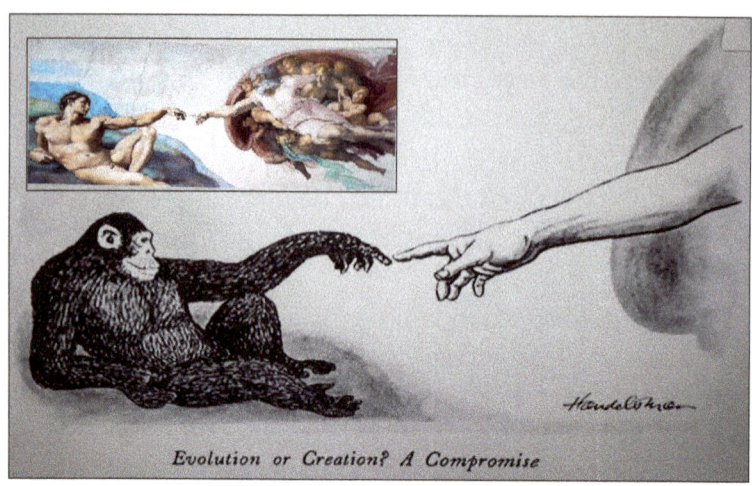

A drawing (reproduced from the New Yorker Magazine, 1989) mocking the Creation Science concept of evolution. The drawing was undoubtedly inspired by Michelangelo's Sistine Chapel painting of God creating man [inset].

---

[5] It is well established that sodium ions, which have a charge of plus 1 (Na^+), are found mainly in extracellular spaces, whereas potassium ions, also having a plus 1 charge (K^+), are found in both intracellular and extracellular compartments.

[6] Ion exchange chromatography is a well-known laboratory technique that is often used to separate organic or inorganic compounds based upon their differences in charge.

[7] Creation Science advances the concept that species' evolution and the design of biological systems are actions of some form of intelligent being. There is no credible evidence to support these assertions, which is advanced as an alternative to the Darwinian concept of evolution.

The Hair Affair

Raymond's hair was turning gray during the time we were together at Downstate. I told him that his gray hair (*see photo*) made him more distinguished looking, but he disagreed. He believed instead that graying made him appear older, an unacceptable idea. We discussed that topic on several occasions, and I asked him what color he would prefer his hair to be.

"I want the color to be black, jet black!" he said.

I countered that jet black would be an unnatural shade. So did his hairdresser. These admonitions did not deter him from dying his hair 'jet black'.

The hair color choice was a mistake that must have been apparent to him the first time he stared at himself in a mirror. He showed up at work for a single day immediately after the coloring change, but then he was not seen again for several weeks.

During his absence I learned that he'd tried to remove the black color altogether, but the color reversal process left him with orange colored hair, not the desired result.

To mitigate this embarrassing situation, he tried dying his hair other colors in the hope of achieving an acceptable tint, but that too was unsuccessful. The failures led him to 'wait-it- out' at home until things had normalized. When he finally returned to work weeks later, his hair had grown out and he once again appeared as he had before, only now he was grayer than ever.

About one year after the hair dying debacle, I left with my family for a sabbatical in France, and during my absence, Damadian resigned his position at DMC and founded FONAR, an acronym standing for 'Field Focused Nuclear Magnetic Resonance' The company would be located in Melville, Long Island.

I did not see or speak to him for several years after he left DMC, but I did follow his progress, even to the extent of buying a few shares of Fonar stock after it began trading on the NASDAQ exchange.

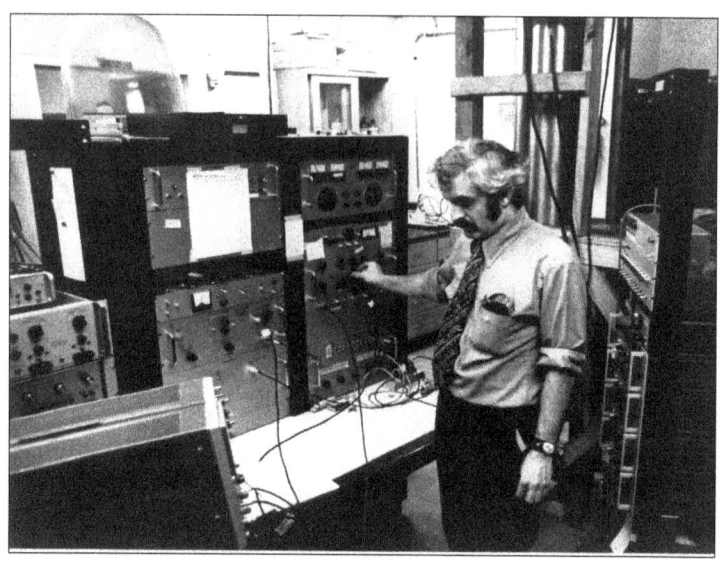

Damadian built his first NMR imaging device at SUNY Downstate. The apparatus included a long cylinder that extended through the ceiling to the floor above. Its imaging chamber was large enough for small animals (e.g., mice).

The 2003 Nobel Prize in Medicine

By 1970 Damadian had identified NMR signal differences between cancerous and normal tissue, and the following year he published his findings. In 1972, he was awarded the first patent for NMR imaging, and in 1976 he reported in the journal *Science* that he had imaged a tumor in a live mouse (*see figure p.21*). Unfortunately, the mouse, which he had named *Pioneer Mouse 1*, did not survive the procedure.

In 1977, Fonar manufactured an MRI scanner powered by a super-conducting magnet made by winding several miles of niobium-titanium wire. The magnet was positioned around an

14

imaging chamber that was large enough to contain a human being. He named this apparatus *Indomitable*.

Years later, he attributed the development of his scanner to *"God's gift...that I got 30 miles of wire at 10 cents on the dollar the instant I needed it is proof that it was God's intention to produce this scan for the benefit of mankind."*

Since no one else in his group was willing to risk being the first human to be imaged in Indomitable, Damadian himself was the first test subject. That attempt was unsuccessful in terms of producing an acceptable image, but at least he suffered no harmful effects from the procedure. It fell to his associate, *Larry Minkoff (photo),* to become the first human imaged in *Indomitable* which was the first MRI scanner to be marketed by Fonar. It differed significantly from the liquid helium-cooled super-conducting

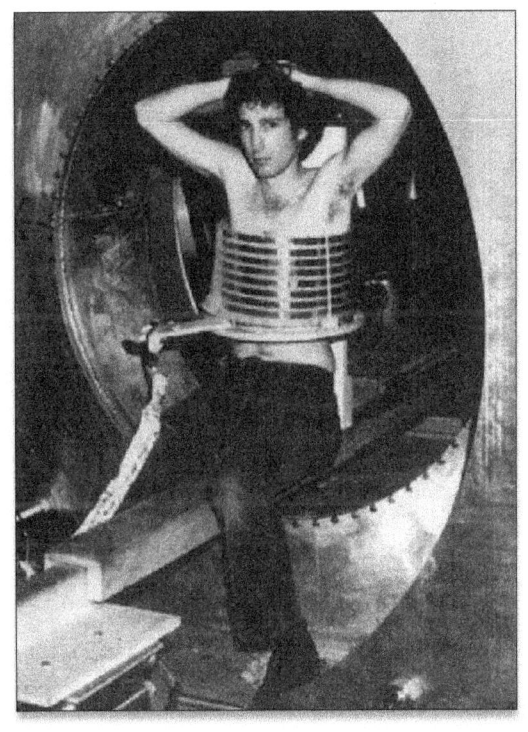

magnetic scanners that were being produced by *General Electric* (GE).

For one thing, the iron core Fonar magnet did not require helium cooling, a feature that permitted greater flexibility in chamber design and size. Unlike the GE MRI chambers, Fonar's chambers were suitable for scanning upright human subjects. Later, they built room-size chambers that permitted real-time imaging of procedures being carried out by a surgeon. In 1997, Fonar won a $129 million judgement against GE for patent infringement.

In 2003, the Nobel Prize in Medicine or Physiology was awarded to *Paul Lauterbur* (University of Illinois and the Brookhaven National Laboratories) and *Sir Peter Mansfield* (University of Nottingham, England) for their work on NMR. Damadian was shut out from this award, and he was infuriated. [8]

---

[8] This is not the first time that candidates worthy of sharing the prize have been excluded. In 1962 *James Watson, Francis Crick, and Maurice Wilkins* were awarded the Nobel Prize in Physiology or Medicine for their discovery of the structure of DNA. *Rosalind Franklin's* X-ray diffraction pattern was the key evidence for developing their model. Her contribution was not acknowledged by the awardees. In any event, Franklin was not eligible for the prize-she died four years before the award was made. Reportedly, the Nobel awardees acknowledged the importance of her work several years later. Another example of exclusion from the Nobel Prize involved *Chien-Shiung Wu*, whose 1949 discovery of 'parity laws' were critical discoveries that led to the 1957 Nobel Prize award in Physics to *Chen Ming Yang* and *T.D. Lee* for their own investigations of parity laws. In his Nobel lecture that year Yang *(cont. p22)*

To express his displeasure, he took out full page ads in The New York Times, The Los Angeles Times, and other major newspapers. These ads featured an upside-down image of the Nobel Prize medal followed by a vituperative and disparaging narrative (*see below*).

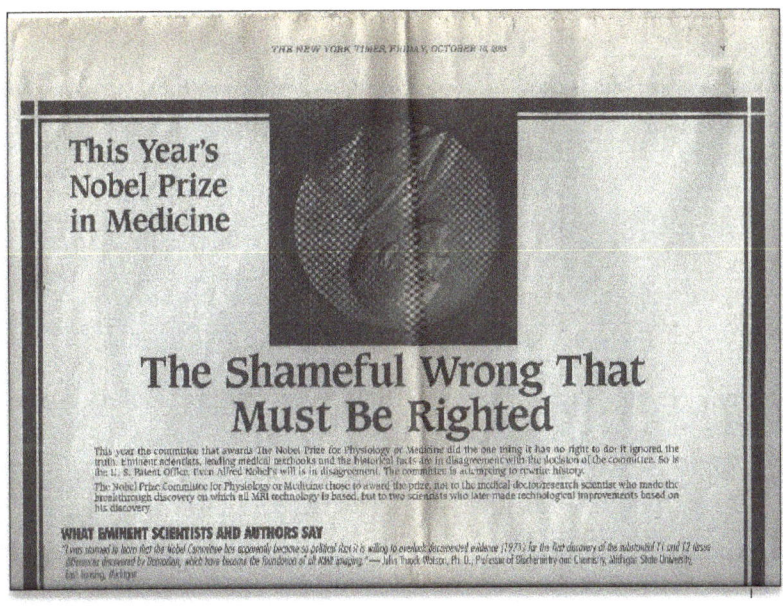

(cont. from p21) acknowledged how crucial Wu's experiment had been for their success and Lee later pleaded with the prize committee to recognize Wu's contributions. These sentiments were echoed by other qualified scientists, to no avail. Wu's related work on quantum entanglement between 1949 and 1971 provided an experimental basis for awarding the 2022 Prize to *Alain Aspect, Anton Zellinger,* and *John Clauser* for 'experiments with entangled photons.' By the time that award was made Wu had died.

His displeasure was also chronicled in an article in *Smithsonian Magazine* which documented his important role in the development of MRI scanners. Despite many public protestations and presentations, publication of newspaper ads such as the one above, magazine articles, and requests from colleagues to the Nobel Committee, there was no response from the Nobel Prize Committee, and to be sure, there was no change in their decision. It is not clear why Damadian was excluded from the prize, but among other things, it was related to his partnering with Creation Science.

When I learned that Damadian had been passed over for the Nobel Prize, I contacted him to offer my commiseration. I even paid him a visit at the FONAR facility in Melville during one of my trips to use the Scanning Transmission Electron Microscope (STEM) facility at The Brookhaven National Laboratory. After that meeting, and after having reviewed all relevant information about his qualifications for the award, I sent a personal letter to the Nobel Prize Committee in support of his deservedness for the award, and then another letter to some of my associates requesting that they also support Damadian's quest (*below*).

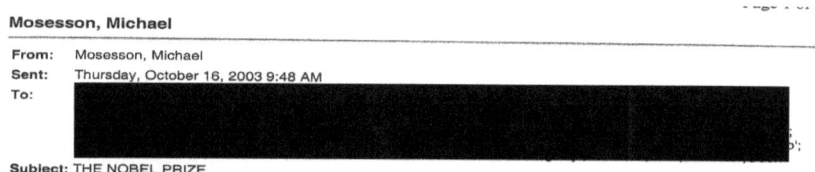

Mosesson, Michael

From:	Mosesson, Michael
Sent:	Thursday, October 16, 2003 9:48 AM
To:	

Subject: THE NOBEL PRIZE

Dear Friends:

    I believe strongly that Raymond Damadian should have been awarded the Nobel Prize this year for his discovery of NMR imaging. I was a close colleague of his for several years at SUNY-Downstate in the 60's and 70's and had the opportunity to observe his experiments and discuss them with him and his coworkers. I have carefully reviewed the relevant literature and patent law, and I believe that it clearly suports Raymond Damadian's position. It does not appear to me that there is much to be done after the fact, but if you feel as strongly as I do about this, you might write to the Nobel Committed directly. The e-mail address is secr@mednobel.ki.se .

Sincerely,

Michael Mosesson

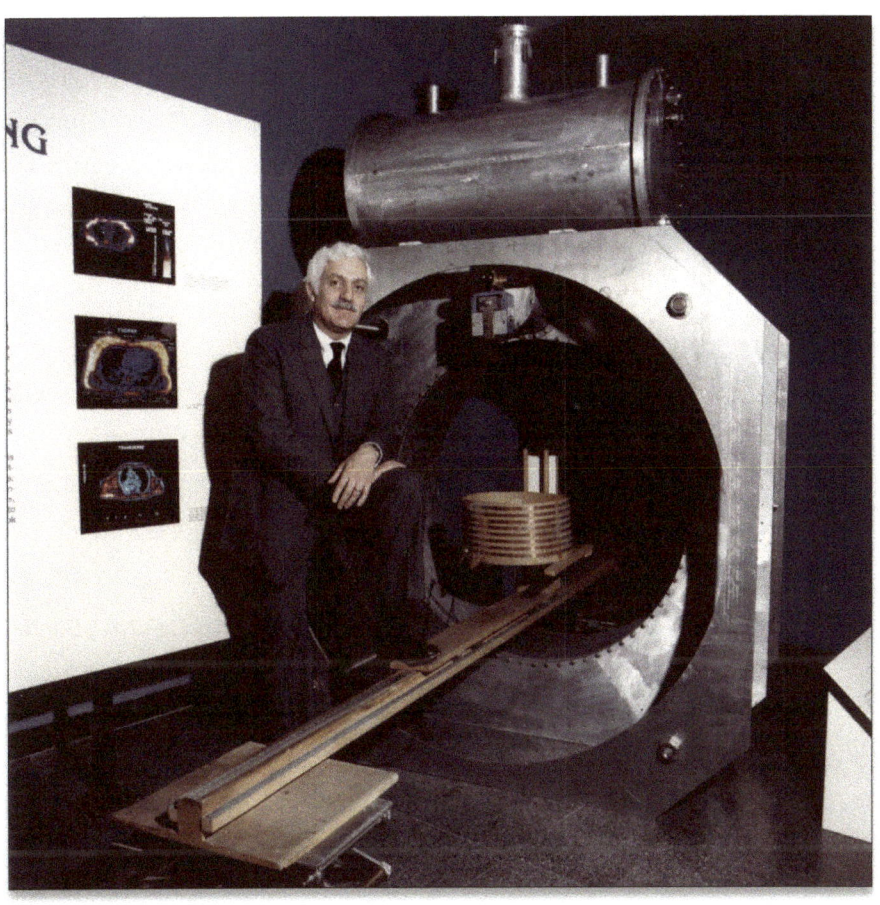

Raymond V. Damadian posing with 'Indomitable', the first whole-body MRI scanner (circa 1989). Indomitable has been on display at the Smithsonian Hall of Medical Sciences. (Reproduced with permission of FONAR Corporation)

Afterword

The rationale for Raymond Damadian's unswerving belief in creation science has always escaped me. Nor have I been able to resolve the disparity that exists between creation science canons and evidence-based scientific discovery.[9] Nevertheless, he was successful in designing an MRI scanner even though he chose Intelligent Design to explain the basis for this and other discoveries. Whether or not Damadian deserved a Nobel Prize remains unresolved, but his achievements will stand in perpetuity.

Michael Mosesson

---

[9] During the course of my research, and teaching career, which spanned more than 55 years, I have personally encountered or been associated with scores of scientists, pre- and post-doctoral students, educators, and four Nobel Laureates, including *Christian Anfinsen* (for work on *Ribonuclease*), *Marshall Nirenberg* (for deciphering *The Genetic Code*), *Stanley Prusiner* (discovery of *Prions*), and *Robert Furchgott* (for his work on *Nitric Acid as a Cellular Signal*). Furchgott was a revered teacher of mine (Pharmacology) when I was a medical student, and years later, a faculty colleague at DMC. To my knowledge, none of them has given credence to the concept of intelligent design.

Chapter 3
THE MILWAUKEE HEART PROJECT
A Tale of Success and Failure

The renowned Milwaukee thoracic surgeon, *Robert J. Flemma*, burst into my office one day in the Spring of 1986 without knocking. It was my first meeting with this robust and outgoing man, and he got right to the point.

"I want to build a totally implantable artificial heart," he said, "and I want you to help me do that."

That introductory remark was followed by several minutes' worth of formal introductions and background information before we returned to the subject of the artificial heart.

It was clear that Flemma had been conjuring up this project for some time and had already figured out how it would be conducted. He would be one of a triumvirate of directors and would contribute to surgical aspects of the project. He also mentioned other initiatives that were outside the scope of the heart project, such as developing an operative procedure called *'cardiomyoplasty'*.

In addition to his surgical skills, Flemma had other qualifying bona fides. During his professional career he had co-authored a few clinical case reports or clinical studies concerned with cardiovascular surgery. Just as important, he intended to donate money from his own resources and help raise additional funds from sources in the Milwaukee community.

The second member of the triumvirate would be his close professional associate, *Donald H. Schmidt*, who headed the Cardiology Section of the UW Medical School's Milwaukee Clinical Campus at Sinai Samaritan Hospital. Schmidt would be in charge of experimental animal aspects of the Heart Project, primarily through his associate in the Cardiology Department, *Carl Christensen*, PhD.

Schmidt was a competent clinician and administrator. He had graduated from The University of Wisconsin Medical School and then undertook post-graduate clinical training at Columbia University Medical Division at Bellevue Hospital in New York City. His post-doctoral training was interrupted by several years of military service in Germany during The Cold War. Following that stint he returned to New York and completed cardiology training at Bellevue Hospital.

Shortly thereafter, *Richard Rieselbach*, Dean at The Milwaukee Clinical Campus of the University of Wisconsin Medical School, recruited him to head its Cardiology Section. A few years later, Rieselbach would recruit me to be Director of The Research Division and Co-chairman of the Department of Medicine.

Given my expertise in thrombosis and hemostasis, it seemed inevitable that I would be brought on board as the third director. Most importantly, I would be responsible for hematological/cell biological research and development, an aspect of the project that included the daunting task of rendering *luminal* device surfaces (i.e., inner surfaces coming in contact with flowing blood) *'non-thrombogenic'*[10].

Secondly, my participation as Director of The *Winter Research Institute* (WRI) was necessary. This facility contained ample laboratory and office space plus a fully accredited Animal Care Facility that would be used for evaluating implanted heart devices in experimental animals.

---

[10] 'non-thrombogenic' means minimization of the potential for thrombus (blood clot) formation.

At the inception of the MHP in 1986, my laboratories on the third floor of the WRI included a state-of-the-art electron microscope facility. The Animal Care Facility on the second level would also provide space for a machine shop where devices designed, assembled, and bench tested. *In toto,* the WRI was an ideal institutional resource for carrying out the project.

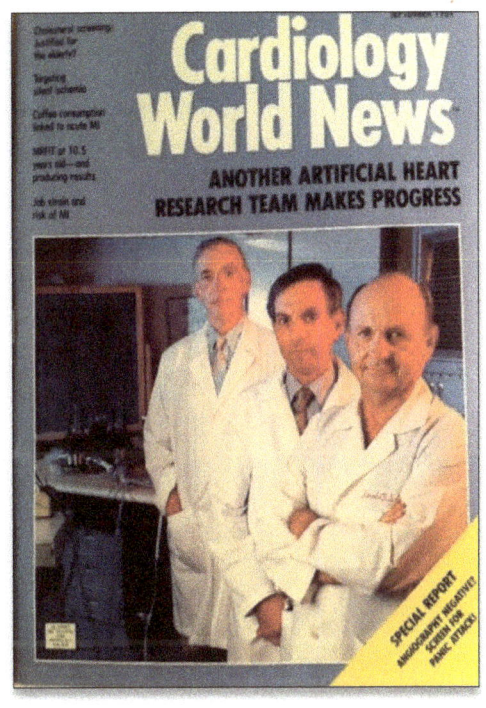

In the weeks that followed our agreement to launch the MHP, we discussed many aspects of the forthcoming initiative. Flemma made clear his intent to donate money of his own and he was confident that he and Schmidt, both of whom had considerable clout with affluent members of the Milwaukee community, would raise considerably more.

We also discussed recruiting *Michael J. Cudahy* to become chairman of The Board of Directors. Cudahy was a well-known Wisconsin businessman and philanthropist, and the president of Marquette Electronics, a medical electronics and devices company. Cudahy would help to populate the Board with prominent members, including *Bob Abdoo (Wisconsin Electric CEO), Gary Grunau (Grunau Construction Company), Charlie McNair, John Galanis, and others.*

Other recruitments included *Bob Uecker*, the revered announcer for The Milwaukee Brewers baseball team, who would help us raise money by lending his name to golf tournaments, and other fundraising events that occasionally included movie stars like *Cindy Crawford (right)*.

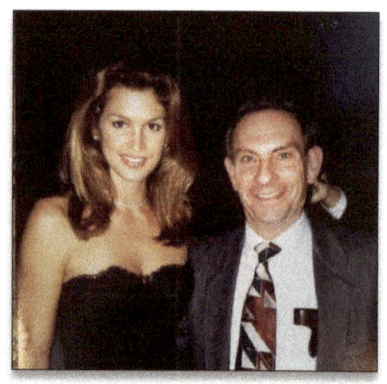

Cudahy eventually donated several hundred thousand dollars to the project. We also received contributions from the University of Wisconsin Medical School. By 1989 we had raised $2.7 million. In addition, the MHP was named as one of five locations endorsed by the federal government to pursue VAD and TAH development. That money spigot slowed significantly after Bob Flemma's death[11] that same year.

I realized at the outset of the triumvirate agreement that my vote could not override those of Schmidt and Flemma who seemed to be 'joined at the hip' in all matters. That led to my misgivings about their ability to handle critical scientific and administrative aspects of the project. One of these items was their refusal to apply for Federal funding; their attitude based upon the mistaken notion that such funding would subvert their efforts to commercialize the project. Ten years later, those misgivings became a reality, as evidenced by Donald Schmidt's refusal to co-sign a Grant-In-Aid funding request to NIH (*vida infra*).

---

[11] Flemma had developed a *dilated cardiomyopathy* and was at The University of Utah Hospital awaiting a heart transplant when he experienced a cardiac arrest. He died a few days later in March 1990 at the age of 55. It is ironic that he had spurred the development of a device that might have replaced his heart had he lived long enough.

Heart Devices at the Inception of the MHP

Christian Barnard, a South African thoracic surgeon, performed the first successful human heart transplantation in 1967. In 1969, *Denton Cooley* from Baylor University carried out the first human heart transplantation in the United States. Cooley was also the first to implant a temporary 'total artificial heart' device in a human subject. That patient, *Barney Clark*, lived for three days with the installed device.

Another heart device, the *Jarvik 7*, was first installed in 1982 at The University of Utah by *William DeVries*. A second implantation of that device took place in 1985. The recipient lived for two weeks before receiving a human heart and he survived for an additional 620 days. After that, Jarvik 7 was used only as a 'bridge' to a human heart transplantation. Clearly, there was room for device improvements at the time the MHP was launched.

Designing the Total Artificial Heart (TAH)
–Thrombogenicity[12]–

My first job after joining the MHP was to assemble a Cell Biology Laboratory group that would investigate the question of device thrombogenicity. In my search for someone to lead that effort I placed an ad in *Science* magazine. There were more than twenty replies. After reviewing them and holding several interviews, I chose *Peter Lelkes*, an Israeli citizen who had been born in Hungary.

During his childhood, Lelkes emigrated to West Germany with his family and became a German citizen where he later earned a PhD in Membrane Physics. He then emigrated to Israel where he spent five years at the Weitzmann Institute in Rehovath working on membrane

---

[12] Thrombogenicity refers to the potential for a blood-contacting surface or structure to support formation of blood clots (thrombi).

biology. Following that he spent four years as a Visiting Scientist in The Laboratory of Cell Biology and Genetics at NIH. His qualifications and background were more than adequate, his letters of reference were exemplary, and I offered him the position which he quickly accepted. Within a few months he and his family had relocated to Milwaukee and began organizing and staffing the Cell Biology Laboratory.

During the first few years, he launched several investigations of the flow characteristics of blood passing through polyurethane bladders with a variety of 'texturized' surfaces (smooth, micro-texturized, rough). The Cell Biology group also investigated proteins such as fibrinogen, fibronectin, or cross-linked gelatin, for their ability to support endothelial cell attachment and proliferation.

Left Ventricular Assist Devices (LVADs)

An LVAD is a blood pumping device that connects the left ventricle of the heart to the aorta to augment cardiac output. The *Sarns/3M LVAD*, a pneumatically driven device (*right*), was provided to the project by *William Pierce* of Penn State University. Flemma and his surgical associates installed these devices. These efforts were skillfully supported by *Carl Christensen*, the director of the Cardiovascular Research Laboratory who also coordinated the studies in

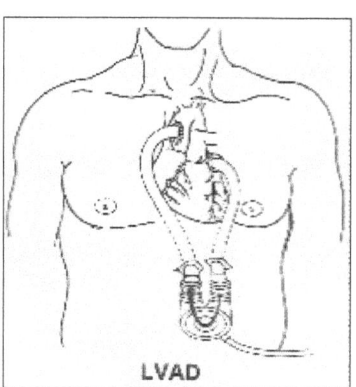

LVAD

Concept drawing of an installed Sarns LVAD

calves. In 1988, after receiving FDA approval, Flemma's associates successfully installed the Sarns/3M LVAD in two human subjects as a bridge to a human heart transplant.

Installation of polyurethane bladders (*right*) was required in LVADs and other circulatory assist devices, to provide a leak-proof conduit for blood passing through the device.

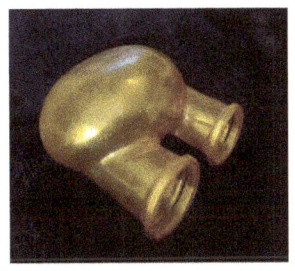

In an effort to determine which type of surface covering was optimal for attachment of vascular endothelial cells, modified surfaces ranging from smooth to micro-textured, were prepared and evaluated *in vitro*. These studies were subsequently extended to studies of calves with an implanted LVAD. *David Amrani*, an associate investigator in my NIH funded Program Project Grant, played a significant role in studying the thrombogenicity of calf-implanted LVADs that had been surfaced with vascular endothelial cells. Amrani also developed and patented a blood test for measuring the thrombogenic potential of implanted devices.

The Total Artificial Heart (TAH)

The project goal was to design and build an implantable battery- powered biventricular device (TAH) that would serve as a permanent replacement for a failing human heart. Safe, long- term survival of human subjects with an implanted TAH required that all *luminal surfaces* of the device (i.e., surfaces or valvular structures coming into contact with flowing blood) be 'passivated' (i.e., non-thrombogenic).

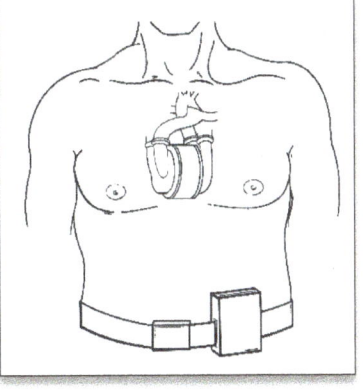

Concept Drawing of The TAH, In Situ

27

Preparing luminal surfaces that were minimally reactive with blood, formation of intra-luminal blood clots (*thrombi*) could be mitigated or even eliminated. Passivation was an unattainable goal in all previous device development projects, and accounted for why none of them, regardless of mechanical design, could remain implanted in the circulation for more than brief periods. Our approach to the problem of biocompatibility was to develop methodology for seeding luminal surfaces with vascular endothelium, have these cells attach firmly to the surface and then grow to confluency. We hoped to use vascular endothelial cells that had been harvested from the adipose tissue of each device recipient, thus eliminating the potential for immunological rejection and inadvertent transmission of blood borne infectious agents.

Mechanical design of the TAH was predicated by the belief that optimal functionality could be achieved by incorporating a motor that operated unidirectionally and that was coupled through a gear reduction system providing individual control of each ventricular chamber. That design plan was initiated and achieved by *Hua Gao,* a thoracic surgeon from mainland China who had come to Milwaukee with the expectation of advancing his surgical skills and knowledge by working with Flemma and his colleagues. These expectations were never realized for reasons that are explained below.

Shortly after completing surgical training in China (1987) Gao wrote to *Robert Flemma* hoping to expand his surgical expertise by working with him and his team. Soon after receiving an encouraging reply from Flemma, Gao came to Milwaukee where he soon applied for accreditation as a surgeon. Gao's request was denied and that prevented him from realizing his stated goals. That denial turned out to be a windfall for the MHP.

Several years before Hua entered medical school, his father was imprisoned by the Chinese government for unspecified reasons. That event left him responsible for supporting his family and caused him to defer his goal of attending medical school. Instead, he worked for several years in a machine shop learning that trade. By the time he completed that stint, he had mastered mechanical engineering, an expertise that later on would serve him and the MHP well.

Although Flemma could not offer Hua the opportunity to improve his surgical skills, he instead offered him the opportunity to join the MHP and work on TAH design. Flemma probably did not fully appreciate Gao's potential as a design engineer and machinist, but he must have understood the value of coupling Hua's engineering expertise with his knowledge of cardiac physiology. Hua accepted Flemma's offer and, as matters turned out, he was almost solely responsible for the design and fabrication of the TAH.

The TAH (Total Artificial Heart)

The TAH (Total Artificial Heart) design was based on the concept that functional efficiency and efficient heat dissipation could best be achieved using an internally installed motor operating unidirectionally and coupled through a gear reduction system for separate control of each ventricular chamber.

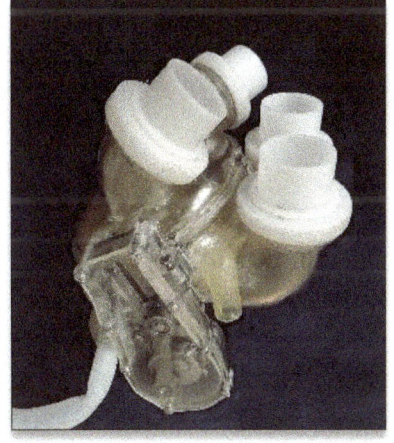

A prototype TAH *(right)* with transparent housing was useful for revealing the gearing that controlled the output of each chamber.

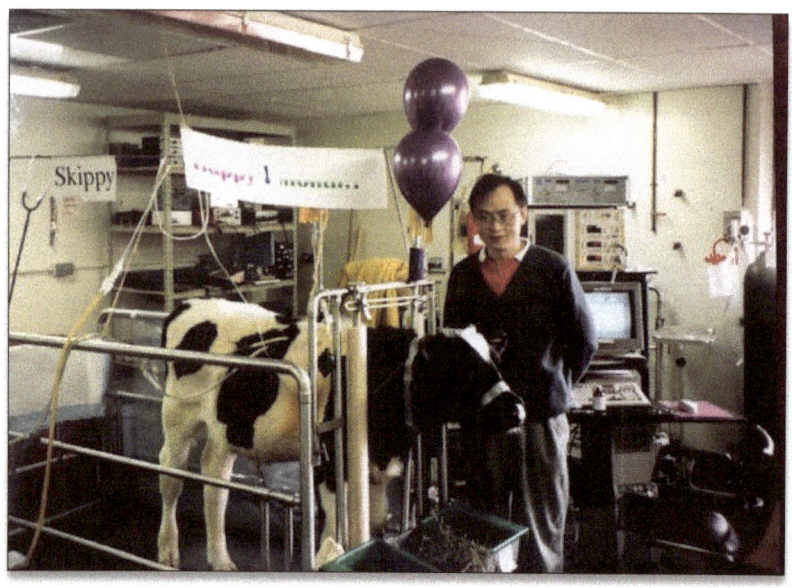

Hua Gao with 'Skippy', the calf that survived for 64 days with an implanted TAH IV.

The TAH went through several iterations of design. The fourth version, TAH IV, was implanted in six-week-old calves to evaluate its potential for long term use. Calves of that age were chosen for study because their chest cavity was the same size as that of an adult human subject. 'Skippy' the calf received TAH IV and survived for 64 days (*above*). Unfortunately, a bearing failure in TAH IV on day 64 led to termination of the experiment.

The final design of TAH V (*below*) eliminated the possibility of bearing failure, a complication that had occurred with its predecessor. TAH V provided a better anatomical fit, exhibited improved hemodynamic function, and reduced heat generation by the internalized motor. The gearing arrangement could increase the left ventricular compression rate and output, while at the same time reducing the output of the right ventricle, a feature that eliminated the need for a compliance chamber. TAH V was tested operationally

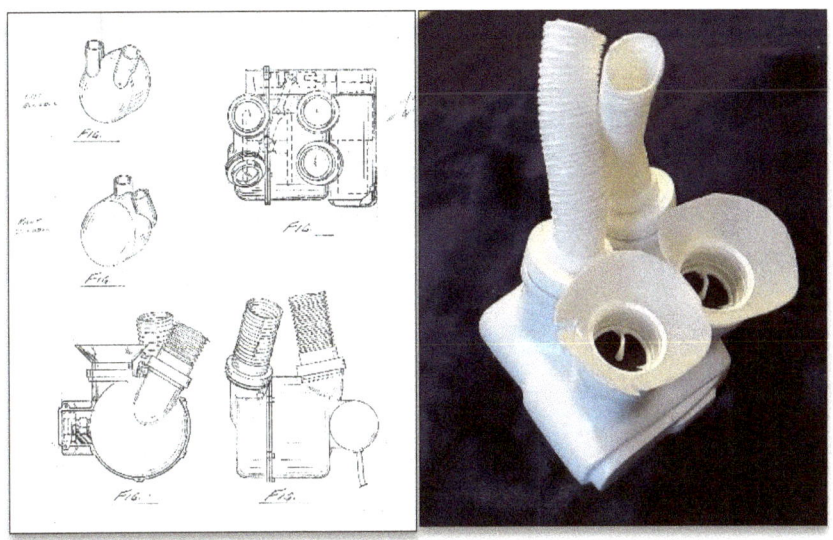

TAH drawing (left) and the TAH V device (right)

in a water tank and performed flawlessly for months.

We were now prepared to carry out additional calf implantations and continue to further refine endothelialization of luminal surfaces. We were also in position to contemplate undertaking human trials of TAH V.

The Demise of the MHP

Following Bob Flemma's death in 1990, fundraising slowed dramatically, and by 1996 the MHP Foundation had exhausted its funding. Aurora had underwritten project expenses for three years to the tune of more than $3.5 million. That situation was about to change.

Since the beginning of the project, *Schmidt* and *Flemma*

had adamantly rejected the idea of seeking or accepting contracts or grants-in-aid from the Federal government (i.e., NIH), ostensibly because of their belief that through 'governmental interference' they would lose administrative control of the project and the potential for commercialization. I believed strongly that these concerns were unfounded, but I could not persuade them to change their view. As stated before, I had had misgivings about not being able to affect such decisions, but I had set them aside. After Flemma's death in 1990 there were just two project directors, but the voting impasse had not changed.

After nearly ten years of enduring their reluctance to apply for Federal funding, plus my realization that the further development and ultimate success of the TAH project was in serious jeopardy, I changed my tactics. Over a period of about two months, I single-handedly organized and wrote a grant proposal to NIH in response to an RFP (Request for Proposals) that targeted development of artificial heart devices. Right up our alley! Shortly after I had completed the grant proposal, I went to Schmidt's office to ask for his co-signature on the application, but he refused. I was deflated by his failure to appreciate how important this grant proposal was for MHP survival. A few months later, Aurora, no longer willing to carry the project's expenses, closed the MHP and dismissed the entire staff. They had been underwriting the project for several years and were no longer willing to continue along that pathway. Since I was not on the Foundation payroll, I was able to remain in place for a few months longer.

In a belated effort to find support for human trials, I contacted several commercial companies, including Medtronics and Baxter Healthcare, but none of them showed any interest in what for them would have been an expensive and problematic undertaking given the absence of a venue and staff. At that time, I was in the process of relocating my activities to the Blood Research Institute (BRI) and would no longer be able to offer the facilities and expertise that had existed at the Winter Research Institute. I could no longer make a credible argument for the project's viability.

I also attempted to relocate what remained of the heart project to the Veterans Administration Hospital (VAH) in Milwaukee, an affiliate of the Medical College of Wisconsin (MCOW). The VAH had an Animal Care Facility that might have served for continuing animal trials, and that could have served as a base of operations for further laboratory investigations. Unfortunately, I was unable to generate any interest in this proposition from the Dean at MCOW. The MHP was now beyond moribund! In 1999, I departed for The Blood Research Institute (BRI) of The Blood Center of Wisconsin.

Afterword

An important project participant, *Luke Smith*, who had been project manager for several years, became a high school teacher. *Hua Gao* initially became a stock market day trader. He then joined *Bradshaw Medical* in Kenosha, Wisconsin and continued his engineering design career. During his stay at Bradshaw Medical he was responsible for 33 patents on orthopedic torque limiting and ratcheting devices.

Carl Christensen moved to Austin, Texas with his wife Kathleen. *Peter Lelkes* obtained a position at Hahnemann Medical School (the Homeopathic Medical College of Pennsylvania). I have heard nothing more about him since his departure. *David Amrani* left my hemostasis research group in 1996 for a position at Baxter Healthcare.

Victor Nikolaychik, an emigree from Belarus (USSR), had been working with the cell biology group on vascular cell endothelialization. For a short while he continued those studies in my laboratory at the BRI. I was not able to offer him salary support and I had limited resources to fund studies on endothelialization. His interest petered out as did my contact with him.

About one year ago, twenty-two years after the demise of the MHP, I began to write a detailed summary of the project with the goal of memorializing its now forgotten successes and failure. I completed that task from notes, memos, and other documents in my possession. I also had several enlightening conversations with *Carl Christensen* who reviewed the manuscript to verify the accuracy of my reporting and description of events that had taken place. Carl also put me in touch with *Hua Gao* who graciously provided documents, newsletters, newspaper articles, and photos concerned with his role in designing and building the TAH.

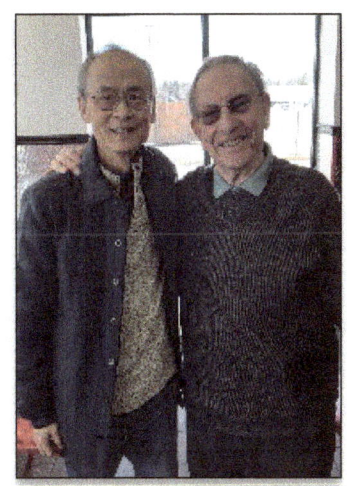

After learning of Donald Schmidt's death in March 2022, I attended his memorial service and spoke with his wife, *Mary Kay Schmidt*. She revealed that Donald possessed many documents and artifacts

Hua Gao and me, May 2022

pertaining to the MHP. A few weeks later, I visited her home to examine the boxes and cartons that contained documents and TAH devices. Mary Kay allowed me to photocopy many of the documents and she gave me one TAH prototype device and one TAH V device. The knowledge that I garnered from these individuals, combined with my own documents and recollections, provided an authoritative basis for compiling this story.

Michael W. Mosesson

Chapter 4

UNDERMINING THE PEER REVIEW PROCESS

Introduction to the process of 'peer review' accompanied the publication of my first scientific report on the preparation of plasminogen-free fibrinogen [1]. I was serving in The Public Health Service (PHS) at the rank of Senior Assistant Surgeon and stationed at The Laboratory of Blood and Blood Products (LBBP) on the NIH campus.

After compiling the experimental parts of my investigation, I turned to *John Finlayson*, my next-door neighbor at LBBP, and asked for his help in organizing, writing and submitting the paper. His help involved most aspects of manuscript preparation and submission, including the process of peer review. He also helped me with writing and organization of the paper, and he graciously insisted that I be the sole author of the paper. Without that help, I would not have experienced the success that I did–the report was accepted for publication shortly after it had been submitted. I had no notion at the time that publishing papers would not always be that uncomplicated

During the three years that I worked at LBBP John helped me in numerous other ways that included working on my writing skills. As a result of the relationship that developed, we collaborated on several research projects, some of which were completed after my tour in the PHS. Later on, even as our individual interests diverged, I continued to request that he review many of my manuscripts. Our friendship endured for more than sixty years until his death in 2022.

Peer Review is the key event at the editorial level for evaluating the 'worthiness' of a submission for publication. Usually, it is the predicate for revision, acceptance or rejection. The process is intrinsically fair, and most often it works as intended. Unfortunately, there are some difficult-to-remediate flaws, especially in its implementation, that can lead to its subversion. The following narrative describes one of those flaws in which I was an unwilling party.

Peer Review

Submitting an original manuscript to a journal for publication involves critical written review and evaluation of its worthiness for publication by reviewers selected by the journal's editors or editorial staff. Reviewer identities are not disclosed to the author, nor is the identity of one reviewer disclosed to another. After reviewers' critiques have been returned, the editor decides whether the article is acceptable for publication as submitted, whether modifications, clarifications, or justifications of one or more of its parts will be necessary for acceptance for publication, or whether it is categorically unacceptable for publication.

Authors are provided with a decision letter from the editor that includes copies of reviewer critiques. In the case of editorial rejection, or when responses or revisions to reviewers' comments are required, the authors may respond in several ways. They may rebut or challenge any or all comments, they may clarify or revise their presentation in response to the critiques, or they may accept the negative editorial decision and offer no response.

The review process is sometimes abused by rogue reviewers who wish to block or delay publication of otherwise valid scientific work, who write biased or unsubstantiated negative critiques, or who even plagiarize the contents of the manuscript while delaying its publication. Despite these shortcomings, peer review remains the method of choice for evaluating scientific investigations.

Mattia Rocco and the Road to Subversion

This section of the narrative describes a unique attempt by my erstwhile friend and former colleague, *Mattia Rocco*, to undermine the peer review process. I was an unwilling party and witness to that attempt.

Rocco earned his PhD at the University of Genova for work that involved the use of physical analytical techniques to model the structure of macromolecules, such as fibrinogen. Rocco later expanded his experience and knowledge with post-doctoral fellowships, or as a visiting scientist in North Carolina, The Netherlands, and California. Eventually, he secured a Staff Scientist appointment at The Advanced Biotechnology Center in Genova.

I first met him at a fibrinogen research conference that took place in Milwaukee in 1988. We met again in Rouen, France, when *The International Fibrinogen Research Society (IFRS)* was founded. In the years that followed, a friendship emerged, highlighted by a visit with my family to his home in Genova.

I was sufficiently impressed with Mattia's scientific qualifications and achievements to write a letter (1993) supporting his application for a fellowship award from the International Union Against Cancer. The fellowship was spent with *Russ Doolittle* at UCSD in California.

From the very beginning of the relationship, I recognized Mattia's tendency to publish his work prematurely. Usually, these studies were peppered with an incomplete understanding of the biological and physiological aspects of the subject he had addressed. Often, he failed to carry out important control experiments, which in turn resulted in problematic interpretations and questionable conclusions. He usually acknowledged these shortcomings but excused his behavior by invoking the pressure he felt to 'publish or perish'.

On one occasion he asked me to review a final 'draft' of a manuscript on *the effect of calcium chloride on the rate of fibrinopeptide release from fibrinogen by thrombin*. I accepted that request and soon provided him with a detailed commentary. My review and the events that subsequently took place are the basis for this story.

In my review of the manuscript, I pointed out flaws in experimental design, the lack of certain controls, and the tenuous interpretations and conclusions that followed from these shortcomings. Nevertheless, shortly after receiving my comments, he submitted the paper to *Blood* for review.

I did not know for sure whether he had made any changes in response to my critique, but the short period of time that elapsed between providing my review and its submission to *Blood* led me to question whether any substantive changes had been made. Any doubts that may have existed were removed when *Sandy Shattil,* the senior editor of *Blood*, asked me to be one of the reviewers. I was beyond curious at that point and accepted his offer.

It was not surprising that I found the submitted manuscript to be nearly identical to the 'draft' version I had recently reviewed. Consequently, the critique that I returned to *Blood* did not differ significantly from my previous review. Although I had faith in the integrity of the peer review process, I nevertheless realized that my identity as 'reviewer 1' would be clear to Mattia since it was so textually close to my original commentary. My recommendation to the editor was that the study design was flawed, lacked adequate controls, and would require revision for it to be acceptable for publication. Not surprisingly, Shattil sent Rocco a letter rejecting the manuscript (*Addendum 1*).

That should have been the end of my involvement in the peer review process, but it did not turn out that way. Shortly after Mattia received the rejection letter he sent me a letter that also contained a copy of both reviewers' critiques that had been interspersed with his own comments (*Addendum 2*). (I underlined some of the text in that letter for easier recognition of parts he had written.). In the first few lines of the letter, he made his intentions clear, namely, to finesse the fact that he was aware that

I had been 'reviewer 1', while at the same time asking for my 'help' as a known 'expert' on that subject.

The second paragraph read:

"I'd like to ask your help, because some *of the major objections we got fall in an area you're definitively the best expert that I know.* Below, I've cut and pasted the rejection e-mail, with some comments of mine in CAPITAL LETTERS, and the manuscript with figures is attached in PDF format. As for where to resubmit it, it may be better to go to a more biochemical/biophysical journal, such as Biochemistry or Biophysical Chemistry. *Your suggestions here will also be greatly appreciated! Mattia."*

Clearly, Mattia had written the letter in anger and frustration and, not surprisingly, showed no interest in addressing any of the issues that had been raised by the reviewers. His interspersed comments were obstinately unaccepting and often sarcastic.

I should not have taken the bait, but my curiosity got the better of me, and I agreed to play his game and perpetuate the fantasy that he was unaware that I was 'reviewer 1'.[13] A few days later, after having worked my way through the annotations, I responded.

October 15, 2002

Dear Mattia:

This exchange is getting out of hand. The discussion is broadening and becoming so diffuse that I can't remember how the discussion evolved in the way that it has. Let me just say that I have by now read your manuscript in detail and can complete my review of it in the context of the two reviewers' comments. That should bring us to some closure on the saga of your FPA manuscript.

Let me start with 'reviewer 2'. His comments are mostly cosmetic and organizational. Most of the points are well taken and should be addressed by you.

41

The point in para 1 about the rationale for the study is very good, and a good reason that the degraded alpha chains in the FPA story should be introduced somewhere.

However, I think that this reviewer knew enough or thought enough about fibrinogen biology to raise the important issues that were raised by reviewer 1.

Now on to reviewer 1: I have to say that I agree with these comments and especially with the suggestions for control experiments, and these recommendations should not be considered to be an option. I also agree with the reviewer that without carrying out FPA release experiments with intact and non-intact fibrinogens, as recommended, and without comparing fibrinogen with and without gamma prime chains, the study would indeed be without good value. The reason for saying that is that the conclusions are too unsupported and tentative to be counted as a definitive advance to our knowledge. If they are published as is, someone else will eventually have to do the controls in order to explain the findings.

I did notice something else about your manuscript that was not raised by either reviewer. Your calculation (Table 2) of ionic strength is wrong and "I.S." is not an accepted abbreviation for ionic strength, which is usually given by a μ or perhaps r/2 (I'm not sure anymore which is preferred, you'll have to look that up). The ionic strength of a solution is not simply the addition of the molarity of the constituents as you have done. The formula is C_i X Z_i squared/2. So the ionic strength of a divalent calcium-containing buffer would be much higher than you have indicated. You also should take into account ionization of the Tris species in the buffer, and that means you have to calculate that using the pK of Tris.

---

[13] The reviewers' critiques and my constructive suggestions did not lead to any meaningful changes in the manuscript, nor did it deter him in the slightest from resubmitting it to *Biochemistry*. What it earned for me was his undying animus and the shenanigans that he perpetrated three years later that I alluded to briefly in chapter 14 of *Fibrinogen Memoirs2*.

Now for a response to some of your latest comments: Your idea that the gamma prime chains CANNOT under any circumstance be responsible for the observations you made is incorrect and your reasoning is wrong. I'm not sure whether gamma prime chains will prove to be responsible for your observations, but they cannot be excluded out of hand as you have done for the reasons you have given. Moreover, I don't know where your idea that they would only affect FPB release comes from.

If you consider the molar content of gamma prime chains in your fibrinogen population, even though they amount to only 10% of the gamma chain population their molar concentration far exceeds that of the thrombin you added, so whatever effect they have on thrombin will definitely be skewed on a molar basis in the direction of binding. Since they have a relatively high affinity for thrombin, since the binding site is not located on thrombin exosite one, there is good reason to believe that this sequence will be reacting with the thrombin early or even at all times, during substrate cleavage, but especially later in the FPA release reaction. The affinity of the gamma prime site approaches that of the substrate site on fibrinogen, but it is at least ten times stronger than the low affinity non-substrate site. So it is not difficult to imagine that as FPA release proceeds, and substrate availability becomes exhausted, the effect of the gamma prime sequence on thrombin activity will become more pronounced. I hope that you can understand this, because if you cannot, we have no easy lines of communication or understanding.

I think as far as the 'fold back' hypothesis is concerned, I don't think that that has anything to do with whether or not the gamma prime chains might or might not have an effect on thrombin release of FPA from fibrinogen, since the gamma prime chains on fibrinogen molecules (or even on fibrin molecules) are not geometrically constrained and can react with thrombin that is binding to any nearby molecule. But since you brought up the subject, I just want to say that you seem to rely totally on crystallographic data (which by the way, cannot speak to the position of the gamma chains, because they could not be visualized in the crystals) and because you have not carefully read or at least considered the experiments that have been published by us and by others, which indicate where the chains must be located in assembled fibrin. Since the crosslinking site on gamma prime chains is the same as on all g chains, it doesn't matter how long the gamma prime extension is. Until you read and fully understand all the experimental evidence from Selmayr to Siebenlist and Medved you will not be able to make a well-reasoned judgement about the crosslinking of gamma chains in fibrin. It is a matter of your being 'stubborn', which you certainly are, but more importantly it is a matter of your being uninformed and unwilling to modify your position.

Mattia, I would like to say that I am not pleased with your unwillingness to accept what the critical control experiments are in your calcium-fibrinogen-FPA story.

The letter exchanges on this matter began in October 2002 and continued until the following March. If it hadn't already been obvious, the pretense that 'reviewer 1' was anyone other than me, had disappeared. Mattia's letters became increasingly vituperative, sarcastic, adversarial, and unfocused, sometimes spilling over to unreasoned and thoughtless criticisms of unrelated work of mine on fibrin cross-linking, about which he understood very little. These exchanges were time-consuming, unproductive and frustrating for me because I was unable to make any inroads on his ignorance, faulty reasoning, or the experimental design and interpretations. By March 2003, I had given up on him and his ideas. I sent one final admonition with a quote by *Samuel Butler*: *"An obstinate man does not hold opinions, they hold him."*

In the spring that year, Shirley and I went on a three week 'Air Safari' tour of the Australian Outback, during which each of the participants piloted their own airplane, in this case a Cessna 172. Each day we would follow-the-leader in a 'conga line' to our next destination. Somehow, Mattia had learned about this trip and written to me, ostensibly to learn more about it.

The letter also contained a section that he had broadcast to all his associates and friends explaining his desperate funding/academic situation and asking for support and ideas on how to navigate such tough waters. In my opinion, his travails related directly to his cavalier approach to science. I responded in detail about our trip but made no mention of his funding problems.

Four months later, after we had returned from Australia, he wrote again to inform me that the manuscript that had been rejected by BLOOD had been resubmitted to *Biochemistry* and had been accepted for publication. He enclosed a preprint of the forthcoming paper, title page reproduced below.

Biochemistry 2003, 42, 12335−12348

12335

Kinetics of Fibrinopeptide Release by Thrombin as a Function of CaCl$_2$ Concentration: Different Susceptibility of FPA and FPB and Evidence for a Fibrinogen Isoform-Specific Effect at Physiological Ca^{2+} Concentration[+]

Aldo Profumo,[‡] Marco Turci,[‡] Gianluca Damonte,[§] Fabio Ferri,[‖] Davide Magatti,[‖] Barbara Cardinali,[‖] Carla Cuniberti,[⊥] and Mattia Rocco*[‡]

U.O. Biologia Strutturale, Istituto Nazionale per la Ricerca sul Cancro, Genova, Dipartimento di Medicina Sperimentale, Università di Genova, Genova, Dipartimento di Scienze CCFFMM and INFM, Università dell'Insubria a Como, Como, and Dipartimento di Chimica e Chimica Industriale, Università di Genova, Genova, Italy

Received March 17, 2003; Revised Manuscript Received August 18, 2003

The title was identical to the one submitted to *Blood*. Except for adding a few literature citations there were no changes in the text, the experimental design, and the flawed interpretation and discussion. The date of its submission to *Biochemistry*, March 17, 2003, corresponded temporally to the letter he had sent while we were on our Australia trip. He made no mention in that letter of having resubmitted the manuscript.

To make matters worse, he added a sarcastic and ingenuous statement in the acknowledgement section that left no doubt about my identity as one of the 'two anonymous' reviewers of the *Blood* manuscript.

I could not resist writing to him again and included some underlines for emphasis.

November 5, 2003

Dear

ACKNOWLEDGMENT

We thank R. Cancedda for support, F. Tosetti for help, R. F. Doolittle for help and advice, and E. Di Cera for very useful discussions and suggestions. Thanks are also due to Mike Mosesson and to two anonymous reviewers for their critiques, for suggesting alternative hypotheses, and for pointing out to us some key references.

Mattia:

Thank you for sending me a copy of your recent publication in *Biochemistry*, and for mentioning me so kindly in the acknowledgements section in the same breath as an icon like Russ Doolittle. I congratulate you for your ability to get this paper published, but the truth is, I'm quite disappointed that you went ahead and published an incompletely controlled set of experiments, the promise of doing future control experiments notwithstanding.

One important comment FYI and close attention: I noted that you cited *Maia Moaddell's* paper (ref 81) in relation to a putative calcium binding site on the gamma prime chain. **Please read that paper again carefully.** There is a large conceptual error built into their experimental design that negates every single one of their major conclusions.

Kevin Siebenlist and I previously pointed this out in several of our publications, if you will take the trouble to read them (try T&H 86:1221,2001 for starters). To wit, what they didn't realize (although *David Farrell* knows this now because I spoke with him

46

about it in Birmingham last July), was that factor XIII (yes, factor XIII not just thrombin-activated XIIIa) is an active calcium-dependent enzyme with fibrinogen or fibrin as the substrate. Their so-called "binding constants" were unrealistically high for non-covalent interactions and in fact they were undoubtedly due to calcium-dependent factor XIII- mediated covalent cross-linking of fibrinogen g chains rather than the non-covalent binding between factor XIII and fibrinogen they thought they were measuring. In effect, their results had nothing to do with calcium binding to gamma prime chains at all, at least in my humble but informed view.

You should also consider the potential artefact of using calcium-containing buffers in your own experiments. Your commercially obtained fibrinogen almost certainly also contained significant amounts of factor XIII which, in the presence of calcium ions, would have been merrily cross-linking the fibrin(ogen) in your mixtures while you were busy measuring fibrinopeptide release (fibrin is cross-linked about 8 times faster than fibrinogen and the factor XIII in the preparation cannot be inhibited by NEM). I have no idea of what effect that might have had on fibrinopeptide release, do you?

One last item. I think I've mentioned to you that I thought I had an explanation for your previous results on early fibrin polymerization. My problem at the time I mentioned it was that I hadn't completed my experiments, and I hadn't written them up either, so I had nothing to present to you, and in any case, I wasn't absolutely sure of my results. Well, I still haven't written them up as a manuscript, but at least I have now written an abstract that I submitted to the ISFP for presentation in Melbourne next March—and I'm quite confident of the results. The point you should be aware of here is that <u>PPACK-inhibited thrombin has a profound non-catalytic effect</u> in promoting fibrin in the course of the polymerization (turbidity), and this effect is easily noticeable early in the fibrinogen-fibrin conversion, even at relatively low thrombin concentrations. The same effect would be expected with non-inhibited thrombin, such as in your own experiments, even at the relatively low concentrations you used.

I hope that this information will promote a re- examination of your previous results and perhaps a new and productive dialogue between us. It seems to me that your light scattering system would be more precise and quantitative than the turbidity one I used in my experiments. At least it's a good subject for us to discuss, possibly even in terms of a collaboration. I will send you a copy of the completed manuscript whenever it is ready for submission, and I'll send you a copy of the ISFP abstract after I have finished analyzing all the data that I expect to present in Melbourne.

I hope to go to NC next year for the fibrinogen workshop, but at this point it's not a sure thing. Shirley fractured her hip in a fall last June and is recovering fairly slowly.

Best wishes, Michael

Rocco responded the next day. There was no indication that he understood the importance of my commentaries and he gave no indication that he would do anything substantive to address them. [*Addendum 3*]. I followed up with a brief note that pointed out his lack of understanding of Factor XIII/XIIIa activation, activity, and inhibition, even though I had no expectation that he would recognize their relevance to his own flawed work [*Addendum 4*]. After that the exchanges ended.

Closing Comments

In this chapter I described how I had participated in an event that subverted the spirit and intent of the peer review process. I have long regretted being a party to it. I hope that I have made clear how damaging Rocco's behavior was to the process of honest scientific inquiry and analysis. It is my hope that by exposing this scurrilous behavior, I will deter others from falling into that trap.[14]

Michael W. Mosesson

Literature Citation

1. Preparation and Properties of Human Fibrinogen Free of Plasminogen. *Biochim Biophys Acta* 57, 204-13, 1962

---

[14] Publication of low quality science is far too common, as highlighted in an article by *Andrew Gelman* in the NY Times Science section (November, 2018): *"At this point it is hardly a surprise to learn that even top scientific journals publish a lot of low quality work–not just solid experiments that happen, by bad luck, to have yielded conclusions that don't stand up to replication–but poorly designed studies that had no real chance of succeeding before they were ever conducted. Studies that were dead on arrival. We've seen lots of examples."*

Addendum 1

The Rejection Letter from Blood

"Oct 10, 2002

Dear Dr. Rocco:

Expert reviewers in the field have evaluated your manuscript entitled "KINETICS OF FIBRINOPEPTIDES RELEASE BY THROMBIN AS A FUNCTION OF Ca^{2}: FPA IS CLEAVED AT DIFFERENT RATES, BUT ONLY AT PHYSIOLOGICAL Ca^{2} CONCENTRATIONS, IN TWO FIBRINOGEN SUBPOPULATIONS CHARACTERIZED BY THE EXTENT OF A[alpha] -CHAIN C-TERMINAL DEGRADATION."

Unfortunately, our final decision is that your paper is not acceptable for publication in *Blood*. It was the uniform judgment of both reviewers that the work as presented did not provide the kind of definitive, new insights that are required for further consideration. The reviewers provided comments to you below, and I hope their assessment of the study's strengths and weaknesses will be helpful to you in your further work.

You will appreciate that the number of manuscripts submitted to *Blood* for publication consideration is very high and that the journal can only accept those that receive a high priority rating based on the definitive and novel nature of the findings reported.

I regret the negative decision on this manuscript but thank you for sending it to *Blood* for consideration.

Sincerely,

Sanford J. Shattil, M.D. Associate Editor Blood Journal

c/o Division of Vascular Biology, Department of Cell Biology The Scripps Research Institute"

Addendum 2

October 11, 2002

"Dear Mike,

After the Munich meeting, we wrapped up a manuscript that we had in preparation for some time on our fibrinopeptides release studies, and we quickly sent it to *Blood*, fully knowing that it was really borderline for that journal. Our idea was to give it a shot, and to revert to Thrombosis and Hemostasis if rejected, maybe in time for the Munich special issue (if still planned). In fact, today I got a rejection e-mail from Sanford Shattill, and I don't think we will fight it, even if only one of the referees sounded negative, while the other didn't make any overall comments (or they weren't made available to us, I'll ask Sanford). But, in order to avoid a similar fate when we resubmit it elsewhere (be it Thr Hem or somewhere else, see below).

I'd like to ask your help, because some of the major objections we got fall in an area you're definitively the best expert that I know. Below, I've cut and pasted the rejection e-mail, with some comments of mine in CAPITAL LETTERS, and the manuscript with figures is attached in PDF format. As for where to resubmit it, it may be better to go to a more biochemical/biophysical journal, such as *Biochemistry* or *Biophysical Chemistry*. Your suggestions here will also be greatly appreciated!   Mattia"

Reviewers' critiques plus Rocco's insertions:

Reviewer 1 Comments:

General comments:
The authors have investigated the kinetics of FPA and FPB release in unfractionated human fibrinogen by thrombin. In 2.5 mM calcium-containing buffer (TBC2.5) FP release curves indicated polydispersity, but not in TBC 14 mM calcium or 30 mM calcium.

The effect in TBC2.5 disappeared by adjusting the ionic strength with NaCl to that of TBC30. As an aspect of their investigation, the authors studied the Aa chain composition of the fibrinogen and found that 75% of the Aa chains were somewhat

51

degraded. They then analyzed their TBC2.5 data and found that FPA release data could be fitted as two exponential functions, and further fitted to correspond to the Aa chain composition. From these results they then concluded that there is a calcium-dependent involvement of C-terminal regions of Aa chains in fibrinogen activation. This conclusion was based upon the unverified assumption that the only significant polydispersity in the unfractionated fibrinogen was due to Aa chain heterogeneity. They also assumed that the Aa chain cleavages they observed in the plasma fibrinogen preparation were due to plasmin, and, in fact, they are not.

While the detailed kinetic measurements of FP release are excellent, and reflect the biophysical expertise of the group, the data interpretations indicate an incomplete understanding of fibrinogen biology. The manipulation of the data to fit exponential curves reveals, at best, an apparent association between FP cleavage and Aa chain degradation. The reasoning implicating Aa chains in the process of calcium-dependent FPA release does not take into account all possibilities. Important, if not mandatory, control experiments have been left out. Without these experiments, the study is valueless.

A LITTLE BIT TOO HARSH, ISN'T IT? VALUELESS? IF COMPLETELY IDENTIFYING A MECHANISM SHOULD BE A REQUIREMENT FOR PUBLICATION, THEN THE LITERATURE WILL BE THINNER. WE REPORTED AN INTERESTING PHENOMENON, WE PROPOSED A POSSIBLE EXPLANATION, WE MADE CLEAR THAT WE DIDN'T HAVE TOTAL PROOF!

The logic in approaching their conclusion regarding Aa chains was based upon the assumption that Aa chain degradation is the only event accounting for polydispersity in their fibrinogen preparation. This is surely not the case. In any event, the presence or absence of degraded Aa chains could have been controlled by comparing FP release from fibrinogen preparations with completely intact Aa chains with those that lack intact Aa chains. Such fibrinogen fractions are easily prepared.

EASILY PREPARED???

Furthermore, there is at least one other heterogeneity in the unfractionated fibrinogen preparation, involving the g chains, that seems more likely to be involved in variations in FPA release than the $A\alpha$ chains. It is well known that g' chains bind thrombin whereas gA chains do not, and both types of chains are present in unfractionated fibrinogen. A comparison of fibrinogen containing only gA chains with fibrinogen enriched in g' chains is an obvious control experiment. This experiment has not been considered but would be a very useful addition to the data sets.

IT WAS MY MISTAKE NOT TO INCLUDE A WORD ON THE OTHER POSSIBLE HETEROGENEITIES IN FIBRINOGEN. BUT REALLY I WOULD BE SURPRISED IF GAMMA CHAINS INFLUENCE FP RELEASE! IN FACT, THERE'S AN OLD SCHERAGA PAPER (HANNA ET AL., BIOCHEMISTRY 23:4681-4687, 1984) WHERE THEY MEASURED THE FP RELEASE FROM 3 DIFFERENT FG POOLS, ONE OF WHICH CONTAINED WHAT THEY CALLED GAMMA-57.5 CHAINS, AND THERE'S NO DIFFERENCE IN FP RELEASE!!!! DO YOU HAVE ANY EVIDENCE OF THE CONTRARY?

Specific comments:

1) **Fibrinogen *Aα* chain heterogeneity**. The authors have apparently overlooked the fact that $A\alpha$ chain heterogeneity in human fibrinogen or in plasmin degraded fibrinogen has been extensively characterized. The definitive literature on this subject goes back to the 70's and even before that. It would be instructive to read all or most of these papers and then cite the relevant articles in context with their own findings. Some of these published reports are summarized in author ref 4.

WE GOT THE PLASMIN "KNOWN" SITES FROM RUSS DOOLITTLE, AND IN FACT I HAVE CITED ITS WORKS. THEN I THOUGHT THAT IT WAS ENOUGH, BUT APPARENTLY THIS WAS NOT THE CASE. COULD YOU POINT OUT TO ME ADDITIONAL TRULY IMPORTANT PAPERS IN THIS RESPECT?

2)   P. 18 - By reviewing pertinent literature, the authors will undoubtedly discover that the known *Aα* chain plasmin cleavage sites do not correspond to the ones observed in plasma fibrinogen, and the assignment of cleavage sites on this basis is therefore likely to be in error. Moreover, the failure to be able to assign 8 bands to known plasmin cleavage sites is not at all surprising.

AGAIN, WHAT ARE THE CRITICAL WORKS HERE? BUT IN ANY CASE, I THINK THIS REVIEWER GREATLY EXAGGERATED THE IMPORTANCE OF TRULY IDENTIFYING ALL THE CLEAVAGE POINTS! PERHAPS WE DIDN'T MADE IT CLEAR ENOUGH, BUT OUR POURPOSE WAS TO GIVE A ROUGH IDEA OF WHAT DEGRADATION PRODUCTS WERE PRESENT IN OUR SAMPLES.

Generally speaking, some very pertinent literature goes based upon the assumption that Aα chain degradation is the only event accounting for polydispersity in their fibrinogen preparation. This is surely not the case. In any event, the presence or absence of degraded *Aα* chains could have been controlled by comparing FP release from fibrinogen preparations with completely intact Aα chains with those that lack intact *Aα* chains. Such fibrinogen fractions are easily prepared.

EASILY PREPARED???

Furthermore, there is at least one other heterogeneity in the unfractionated fibrinogen preparation, involving the g chains, that seems more likely to be involved in variations in FPA release than the *Aα* chains. It is well known that *g'* chains bind thrombin whereas *gA* chains do not, and both types of chains are present in unfractionated fibrinogen. A comparison of fibrinogen containing only *gA* chains with fibrinogen enriched in *g'* chains is an obvious control experiment. This experiment has not been considered but would be a very useful addition to the data sets.

IT WAS MY MISTAKE NOT TO INCLUDE A WORD ON THE OTHER POSSIBLE HETEROGENEITIES IN FIBRINOGEN. BUT REALLY I WOULD BE SURPRISED IF GAMMA CHAINS INFLUENCE FP RELEASE! IN FACT,

-

THERE'S AN OLD SCHERAGA PAPER (HANNA ET AL., BIOCHEMISTRY 23:4681-4687, 1984) WHERE THEY MEASURED THE FP RELEASE FROM 3 DIFFERENT FG POOLS, ONE OF WHICH CONTAINED WHAT THEY CALLED GAMMA-57.5 CHAINS, AND THERE'S NO DIFFERENCE IN FP RELEASE!!!! DO YOU HAVE ANY EVIDENCE OF THE CONTRARY?

Generally speaking, some very pertinent literature goes uncited. This occurs in several places in the manuscript, such as in the fibrinogen $A\alpha$ chain polydispersity as pointed out above.
Another example, but not the only one, is the citation of articles relating to FPB release (e.g., Hurlet-Jensen, et al. Thromb Res 27:419, 1982, etc.)

I'VE TRIED TO NOT OVERCITE, BUT I AGREE THAT I MAY HAVE MISSED SOME RELEVANT PAPERS. ANY SUGGESTIONS HERE?

1)   The title of the paper is much too long and the conclusion in the title is unjustified on the basis of the data presented.

OVERALL, I THINK THE MAJOR POINT IS ON THE LACK OF "CONTROL EXPERIMENTS FOR THE "INTACT FIBRINOGEN", I COULD USE YOUR STUFF, BUT I HATE THE IDEA OF "WASTING" IT FOR FP RELEASE STUDIES. THE WAY WE PERFORM THESE "EXCELLENT" KINETIC STUDIES, WE NEED A LOT OF MATERIAL (3 X 1.5 MG PER TIME POINT).
OUR INTENTION WAS TO "REVEAL" THIS STARTLING FINDING OF PHYSIOLOGICAL CALCIUM, BUT CLEARLY TOO MUCH ADDITIONAL WORK WOULD HAVE TO BE PERFORMED TO DEFINITIVELY PROVE THIS HYPOTHESIS. WE'RE WORKING ON DEVELOPING A CAPILLARY ELECTROPHORESIS METHOD TO ANALYZE FP SAMPLES, IN ORDER TO DRAMATICALLY REDUCE THE MATERIAL NEEDED, BUT WHO KNOWS IF AND WHEN IT WILL

Reviewer 2 Comments:
Biochemical studies that indicate different rates of FPA release,

depending upon calcium concentration and degree of alpha chain carboxy terminal degradation.

Introduction: A very general introduction to the broad subject of fibrinogen biochemistry, but no rationale presented for studying alpha chain variations relative to FPA release. Since the experiments focused on the relation between FPA release not only at different calcium ion concentrations but also relative to the amount of carboxy-terminal degradation of fibrinogen alpha chains, what was the foundation for this aspect of the study?

WE DID NOT START THE WORK WITH THE INTENT OF STUDYING THE ALPHA CHAINS VARIATION EFFECT ON FPA RELEASE. ONLY LATER, WE DID CORRELATE OUR FINDINGS WITH THIS ASPECT.

Methods: Page 8, "Determination of effective endpoint of the reactions": This portion could be shortened to two sentences and Figure 1 can be eliminated.

Methods: "Fibrinopeptides quantification": This section could be summarized succinctly, using references to published technology, especially reference 38 (Kehl et al.).

Results and Discussion, Figures 2 and 3: The validity of the observations is well-documented in these figures, but the data are better summarized by Table 1. Figure 2 could be put into Methods or omitted.

Results, Figure 4: Labels to indicate alpha, beta and gamma chains as well as degraded alpha chains would be useful.
Table 1, showing the relative proportions of $A\alpha$ chain fragments: Would it not be better to combine some of the minor bands of degraded Aa chains, for example, those representing less than 2% of the total and differing in molecular weight from other chains by 2,000 or less. Since conclusions cannot be drawn relative to fibrinopeptide release from these individual chains, the major point of polydispersity could still be made, without this extensive degree of alpha chain fragment information.

Results, Figure 6, molecular weight determinations of the *Aa* chain fragments: Assumptions are made in order to group the *Aa* chain fragments into various molecular size estimations. It would be better to group these fragments according to defined domain content, according to pre-determined molecular information. After having grouped these fragments, analysis shifts to calcium variations and FPB release, but without insight as to why and how the alpha chain degradation influences the rates of FPA liberation.

THIS rs (*sic*) DISCUSSED AT THE END.

Page 23, last paragraph of the manuscript: This section brings together the concepts of calcium concentration, calcium binding, differential release of FPA and FPB, and the effect of Aa chain degradation on fibrinopeptide release. Some of these concepts should be introduced in the beginning of the manuscript, perhaps leaving out the more general aspects of fibrinogen biochemistry that are not essential to the experiment.

Also, the information regarding calcium binding sites on the *Aa* chains should be utilized beforehand in the analysis of *Aa* chain influences on FPA release. A calcium-binding hypothesis should be prospectively proposed, then tested by these experiments.

OVERALL, THIS DOESN'T SEEM A "REJECTION REVIEW", SINCE IT SUGGESTS WAYS OF IMPROVEMENT. WHAT DO YOU THINK?"

Addendum 3

From: Mattia Rocco [mailto:rocco@cba.unige.it]
Sent: Thursday, November 06, 2003 7:01 AM
To: Mosesson, Michael
Subject: RE: Fibrinopeptides and other stuff.

Dear Mike,

Thanks so much for having, as usual, taken the time to read and comment on my work. Your critiques and suggestions are always welcome, as your knowledge of the field is still vastly superior to mine (and I doubt I'll ever catch up!). However, as you well know, I always retain the "right" to disagree with you, a simple example being those experiments with the purified fibrinogen fractions that you call "controls" and I call "further experiments". After all, one of my main problems has always been to publish too little because of extra care, and it's starting to hurt me badly... so, I couldn't wait to have the complete story, and I went ahead. To tell you the truth, one of the two Biochemistry referees also wondered why we didn't do the experiments with less degraded fibrinogen samples, but apparently, either him or the Editor (Earl Davie) were satisfied with our responses. I also hope that you are satisfied by the formulation of the Acknowledgement, since I took great care in trying to convey the notion that you commented on the manuscript (at least in its former *Blood* version), but you didn't quite endorse it. And, by the way, don't humble you too much!!! Everybody knows you're a reference figure in the field.

Coming to your points, first of all thanks for the info about Ca-binding to the gamma' -chain. In fact, we just mentioned the possibility that it binds Ca2+ in the context of the elusive 3rd high-affinity site, but in any case, its' low amounts make it an unlikely possibility. Instead, I have just received an e-mail by Willem Nieuwenhuizen, to whom I sent also the paper, that points out to two 1981 and 1982 papers where he found that fragment **X** still has 3 high-affinity sites and fragment **Y** has

2 high-affinity sites. I have totally missed those references (the damn fibrinogen literature is larger than the Pacific Ocean!), and I'm waiting on my library to retrieve me the papers before responding to Willem. In our discussion about the putative location of the 3rd high affinity Ca site, I thought that Marguerie had conclusively shown that fragment **X** has 2 such sites, but apparently the final verdict is not out yet. What's your opinion on this subject?

Regarding the possible role of Factor XIII, first I cannot resist but to point out that apparently its' activity in absence of thrombin activation is still a controversial point.... but I don't want at all to enter also this arena, as I'm totally unprepared on the subject! In any case, FXIII vs FXIIIA is a moot point regarding our experiments, as we added Ca and thrombin within a short time of each other, and thus we're always talking about FXIIIa. Instead, we're guilty of omitting to specify in the M&M of this paper that we routinely treat with PCMB all fibrinogen solutions that are going to be utilized in the presence of Ca++, to inhibit FXIII. However, we then dialyze out the PCMB, and I wonder if we have really killed the FXIII. As a partial support of having effectively inactivated FXIII with this procedure, we never saw any aggregation in Ca-containing fibrinogen solution during our light scattering experiments. But you're right that's an interesting point, and surely, we'll do some control experiments. Finally, the "Kaminsky effect". You made very interesting observations, and surely, we'll love to pick up on this, as it can help to explain our previous observations! By the way, Leonid Medved was here 2 weeks ago, and he also presented your new thrombin-fragment E complex. In the light of this info, did you see any relevant conformational change in Fragment E upon thrombin-binding? In any case, at present, we haven't yet resumed experimental work, due to the lack of students and/or postdocs. At the end of this month, we should know if we're getting a PhD student and/or a graduate student, and then we could start again. And I'll definitively love to collaborate with you on this subject, but I'm refraining from promising anything at this point, since I STILL have to do work with your purified fibrinogen fractions (this thing it's haunting me!).

Well, that's all for the moment regarding science. I am instead saddened to read about the new health problem Shirley is experiencing, and I sure wish her a quicker and full recovery. Please, give my best to her, and tell her that I'm sure we'll see each other in Chapel Hill. That's almost my home turf, so you can't avoid coming there!

Addendum 4

Dear Mattia:

Just one response to your note. NEM will inhibit factor XIIIa but NOT factor XIII, so adding PCMB to fibrinogen before treating with thrombin is probably useless as far as generating XIIIa during your FP release experiments in the presence of calcium ions. It's just one more of the uncontrolled for variables in your experiments. I can hardly wait until you do those experiments and clarify this whole issue.

Best wishes, Mike

Chapter 5

EVENTS DURING THE DECLINE OF THE CROSS-LINKING CONTROVERSY

Arguments over the location of cross-linked γ chain bonds in assembled fibrin clots began in the 1980's and lasted more than twenty years before the still unresolved controversy descended from its zenith in 2004 and disappeared from the literature. The sunset lasted until 2020 when I tried to resurrect its memory in the first volume of *Fibrinogen Memoirs*, an effort that was extended in *Fibrinogen Memoirs2*.

I had been one of the main participants in the dispute about the arrangement of cross-linked γ chain bonds in an assembled fibrin clot, and a stalwart proponent of *'transverse'* bond positioning. The issue boiled down to one of two arrangements: Either the bonds were positioned *linearly* along each strand of a double-stranded fibril (Fig. 1), or they were positioned *transversely* between fibril strands. (Fig. 2).

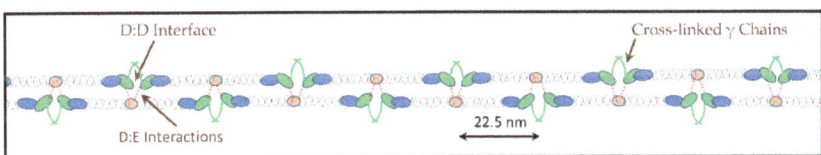

Figure 1. Schematic of a two-stranded fibril with the cross-linked γ chain bonds ⋀ *positioned between the fibrin molecules of each strand.*

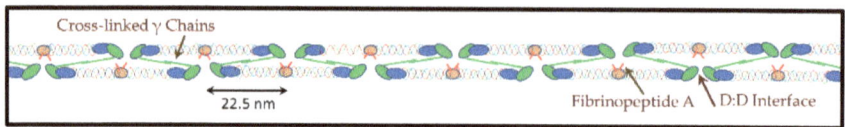

Figure 2. Schematic of a two-stranded fibril with cross-linked γ chain bonds bridging 'transversely' ___ *between the strands.*

In my effort to revive the now moribund issue, I wrote about the cross-linking controversy in both volumes of *'Fibrinogen Memoirs'*. The first iteration was a chapter entitled, *Fibrin, The Perfect Bioelastomer*. The second, cross-linking was the sole topic in *Fibrinogen Memoirs* 2, appropriately subtitled *The Rise and Fall of the Fibrin Cross-linking Controversy*.

Both narratives covered the dispute's history from its beginning through its ascendency, its zenith, and its decline. Not only did I review evidence for each proposed cross- linking scheme, but I also included an assessment of their probative values.

In both books I emphasized the mountain of evidence for a *transverse* bond arrangement, and the questionable evidence for a *linear* bond arrangement. More importantly, I introduced the idea that only *transverse* bond positioning could account for the *elastic* properties of cross-linked fibrin clots. I reinforced that concept by further showing that an *ineluctable* relationship exists between the *transverse* bond arrangement and *fibrin elasticity*. Finally, I added an admonishment: Failure to consider the functional implications of a *transverse cross-linked* bond arrangement would inevitably hamper future interpretation of biophysical experiments.

It might be argued at this juncture that everything worth saying about the cross-linking controversy had been said. Nevertheless, there are some as yet untold tales worth chronicling.

An Event After Publication of the Cross-linking Debate

The cross-linking dispute went on for two decades without ever reaching consensus or resolution. In 2003 *Robert Ariens*, then an Associate Editor of The *Journal of Thrombosis and Haemostasis (JTH)*, suggested that *John Weisel* and I, the main protagonists, formally debate the issue in written articles to be published in JTH. Weisel would present his side of the dispute and I the obverse, *'transverse'*. There would also be opportunities to rebut each other's presentation. That offer was an irresistible opportunity for me as well as for Weisel.

The articles were published in 2004 under the heading: *The Fibrin Cross-Linking Debate: Cross-Linked Gamma Chains in Fibrin Fibrils Bridge 'Transversely' Between Strands.* Naturally, I argued for a 'transverse' cross-link bond arrangement and Weisel argued for a 'longitudinal' arrangement. I felt comfortable in the expectation that the controversy would survive for at least a bit longer.

A few months after the debate articles were published, I met with *Paul Bishop*, a scientist at *Zymogenetics* whose work on commercialization of Factor XIII was widely acknowledged. At our meeting Paul told me about a novel experiment that he had designed that could unambiguously distinguish between the two cross-linking schemes. Although I did not believe it was necessary to carry out additional experiments to prove my case, I welcomed Bishop's idea because it involved electron microscopy that could be carried out by either Weisel or me. Parsing that technicality to Weisel would be an opportunity for a collaboration that, if successful, might resolve the dispute once and for all.

With that outcome in mind, I called John Weisel, discussed the experimental details, and suggested that critical preparative and analytical procedures could be carried out in his laboratory. He agreed to this arrangement and the project got underway shortly afterward [specific experiments are detailed in *Fibrinogen Memoirs 2*].

During the next few months, the project advanced to the final electron microscopic analyses. After several weeks had passed without any communication between us, Weisel abruptly withdrew from the collaboration. On September 28, 2006, he wrote:

"Dear Michael, I'm very pleased to hear that you would be interested in giving a seminar here. The topic should be of interest to people here. I have talked with Krish, who has charge of the seminar series to see what will work best. I'll let you know after I hear back from him.

I am not ready to give up yet on our crosslinking experiments, but the difficulties discouraged Irina in my lab, and we have had too many other things to do. Since this project is not related to our funded research, it has been hard to keep it moving with all the problems we have had."

I did not learn about any results he may have obtained in preceding months, and I never found out exactly what specific difficulties they had encountered. The letter marked the end of the collaboration. I completed my scheduled seminar visit to Philadelphia, but while I was there, we did not discuss any findings he may have made or about the difficulties he may have encountered. And we have not spoken or communicated again about the controversy. I believe that termination of the collaboration contributed to the subsequent decline in attention to the controversy that followed.

A Dustup with the 'Court Jester'

Several months after the collaboration with Weisel had ended, there was another IFRS workshop conference (2006). Because of my concerns for Shirley's health at the time, I did not attend. Shortly after the conference had ended, I received a letter from John Weisel that *Mattia Rocco (right)* had proposed a 'vote' among the attendees concerning which cross-linking hypothesis was correct.

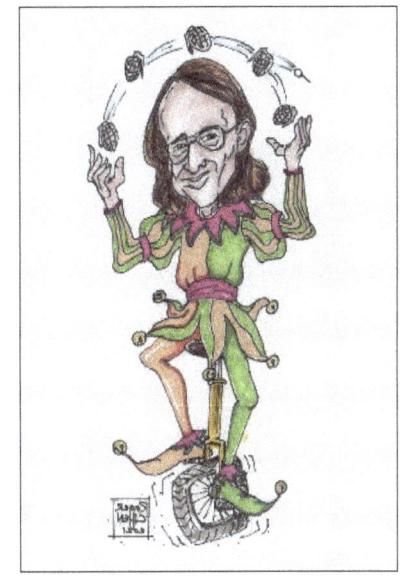

Rocco caricatured as a court jester. (reproduced from Fibrinogen Memoirs2 with permission)

He wrote, *"Johannah is doing all right. How is Shirley doing now? <u>Mattia Rocco dared me to tell you that since you were not at the Fibrinogen Workshop, we had a vote and transverse crosslinking lost</u>. I thought that you would appreciate the humor.*

Best wishes, John"

As previously stated, I had developed a friendship with *Mattia Rocco* at the same time that I attempted, scientifically speaking, to get him tracking in the right direction (see chapter 4). I was aware that he was a Doolittle acolyte who had mindlessly accepted Doolittle's erroneous conclusion that the crystal structure of D-Dimer fragments constituted evidence for a *'longitudinal'* fibrin cross-linking scheme.

It came as no surprise that Rocco would put his ignorance on display at the IFRS workshop by promoting a *'vote'* on fibrin cross-linking schemes. In addition to what he had gleaned from Doolittle, he knew little else about the evidence relating to that subject. I viewed his behavior as cowardly and vindictive and was sufficiently angry to confront him in a letter.

"September 29, 2006

John Weisel told me about you daring him to tell me about your comment at the Fibrinogen Workshop regarding the vote on fibrin-cross-linking. I did not find that comment to be very amusing and I failed to derive any humor from it.

Rather, I found it to be an arrogant and thoughtless gesture to pose that to me as a dare. If you believe that the truth about scientific opinions can be settled simply by a vote, that would confirm my present opinion about the depth of your knowledge and understanding of fibrin physiology and structure. I honestly believe that you have not carefully examined each of the several published and well-documented experiments upon which my opinion on the cross-linking matter is based (including John Ferry's experiments and opinion), or alternatively, that you are not capable of, or willing to, try to understand them. I further believe that you have simply jumped on the crystallographers' band wagon without understanding the fallacy of the argument on the putative relationship between cross-linked D-dimer structure and the cross-linked structure in fibrin.

A few days later I received his reply.

"October 3, 2006

I am deeply sorry that you are upset with me. I have written to John to know more about what happened, and apparently, he wrote you an e-mail, it was not a direct conversation. It is quite likely, then, that the correct setting and meaning of the "joke" failed to reach you (I think that John will also write to you about it). There was absolutely NO disrespect of your work, it was just a lighthearted joke, and the other people around me when I said it apparently thought that it was funny. Had you been around, we would have probably made a joke about Russ (Doolittle), like voting that the crystal structure is wrong...In any case, I did not "dare" John to tell you my joke, I encouraged him to tell it to you (I meant in person), because I was sure you would have found it funny, for what I know of you. I surely hope that next time we'll meet we'll laugh about it over a beer!"

Concerning the "controversy" itself, I have NOT a firm opinion about it, because I didn't follow it closely, I didn't have the time to dwell deeply into it since I'm not working directly on it. It is true, however, that I find it difficult to reconcile your conclusions (I never closely examined your or John Weisel's data, for that matter!!!!) with what the crystal structure seems to tell us, provided that the conformation of fibrin into the fibrils is the accepted rod-like one. The pull-out hypothesis would surely help to reconcile the two datasets, but it seems to me **that at the moment it is just a hypothesis, and** *I would surely love to see it tested. For instance, one could raise antibodies against a recombinant gamma module without that beta-strand, prove that they bind were the pulled-out beta-strand would normally reside, show that they don't bind to fibrinogen, and see if they instead do react with polymerized fibrin (fibrils or fibers). Leonid Medved could surely do this kind of work. Believe me, Mike, I'm just an external observer about this issue, not a player!"*

Among the many things that revealed his ignorance, Mattia dismissed the importance of *Leonid Medved's* 'pullout hypothesis'. He wrote, incorrectly, that Medved's work was *'still a controversial point'*, while in the next sentence he pleaded ignorance of that subject.[15] Although I wrote to him once more, the first letter (above) signaled the end of our relationship. What had once been a well-meaning effort on my part to help him mature as a scientist no longer existed.

Rocco's 'dare', per se, was trivial as far as the cross-linking controversy itself was concerned, but it did reflect the pervasive antipathy to the truth that had developed.

Michael Mosesson

---

[15] *Leonid Medved* and coworkers' experiments leading to the 'pull-out hypothesis' were sound. Their hypothesis stands as one of the pillars in the argument for a *transverse* cross-link bond arrangement, but it does not stand alone.

Chapter 6

JIM MARONEY, AN AVIATION LEGEND

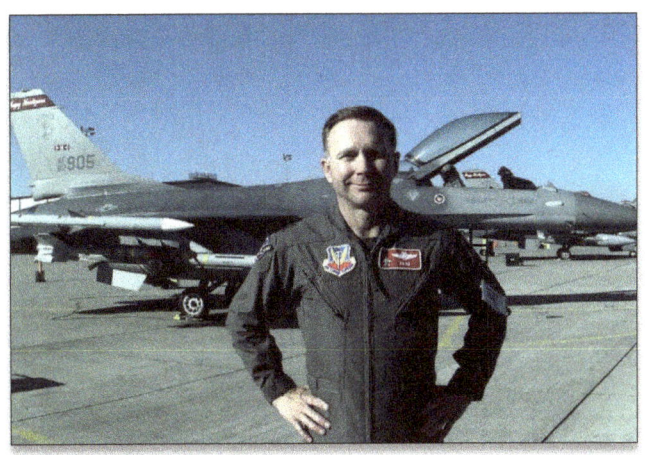

By 1998 the affiliation between Sinai Samaritan Medical Center (Aurora) and The University of Wisconsin was in disarray, and that situation soon further devolved to affect The Milwaukee Heart Project (MHP). Aurora, which had been underwriting MHP activities for almost two years, to the tune of more than two million dollars, cancelled that support, fired everyone working on the project, and shut down MHP operations at The Winter Research Institute.

Over the preceding twelve years, the MHP group had successfully developed a battery-driven implantable biventricular 'total heart' device (TAH) that was shown to maintain a calf's circulation for more than two months (see chapter 3). Despite this success we (i.e., the still living project directors, Donald Schmidt and me) were not able to find financial support for the project's next phase—human clinical trials!

It was clear that my days as The Winter Research Institute director were numbered. In July 1999 I resigned my University of Wisconsin (UW) appointment and transferred my research

71

operations to the Blood Research Institute (BRI) of The BloodCenter of Wisconsin. In return for my years of service to UW, I was awarded an emeritus professorship and a captain's chair with a plaque engraved with my name. A few months after I had relocated to the BRI, I donated the chair to the Mosesson Library at the BRI.

After spending two years in that new position, I was introduced to *Jim Maroney* by his wife, *Susan Maroney*, who, at that time, was a post-doctoral fellow in *Alan Mast's* laboratory. Susan and I had discussions concerning scientific subjects, but when she learned that I was a pilot she insisted that Jim and I meet, and that's exactly what happened!

Jim Maroney earned a BS degree in mechanical engineering at The University of California-Fresno, and shortly afterward, he enlisted in The US Marine Corps to pursue his longstanding interest in a flying career. He went to The Naval Flight Training School and graduated first in a class of 1,500 in 1981. Two years later, he ranked first at the 'Top Gun' Naval Training Weapons School. (As an aside, years later he was a key advisor to *Tom Cruise* during the filming of the movie 'Top Gun').

Maroney continued serving in the Marine Corps until 1985, when he transferred to the North Dakota Air National Guard where he flew F-16 Falcons. He moved up the command ladder to become a Squadron Commander in 1997, and then Group Operations Commander in 2001. That same year, on September 11 ('9/11')., he led an F-16 fighter squadron in search of enemy aircraft and other potential targets.

Jim began to perform in airshows in 1976 and was best known for his acrobatic performances in his DeHavilland Super Chipmunk. In 1985, while maintaining his appointment in the Air National Guard, he joined Northwest Airlines (now Delta Airlines), where he advanced from 'line pilot' to 'chief pilot', charged with overseeing the activities of 600 Delta Airlines' pilots.

Jim and I became friends after our first meeting, and over the years that followed, our friendship grew closer with each encounter. We met regularly for lunch or dinner whenever Jim was in town. On those occasions, he would regale me with stories about his exploits as a navy fighter pilot, an airline pilot, and an airshow performer. He took me for several flights in the Super Chipmunk, demonstrated his flying skills and even taught me how to fly some challenging acrobatic maneuvers.

We also made many flights in Comanche 9390P, most often sightseeing locally, or for practicing instrument approaches. On two occasions, we flew hundreds of miles in a single day to pursue Jim's search for a backup to his Super Chipmunk.

Sometimes, Susan Maroney and I flew in 9390P to attend one of Jim's airshows. On one memorable occasion we flew to Manitowoc, Wisconsin, to watch his performance. That day, just before Susan and I were preparing to return to Milwaukee, Jim asked me to hold 9390P's airspeed at 115 knots so that he could catch up to us in the Super Chipmunk.

Soon after we had departed, Jim came alongside. He asked me to keep 9390P straight and level so he could perform looping maneuvers above and below us. He then repeated that maneuver in a nearly perfect vortex of loops that lasted until we were back in Milwaukee airspace. What a blissful engagement that was, one that will remain in my memory forever.

Shirley and I often met Susan and Jim for evening meals and delightful conversation. The most memorable evening was at Scotty's Crab House restaurant where we celebrated Jim's birthday. The dinner was served in a suite that had a sash-drawn curtain covering the doorway, a setup that would have existed in a 19th century brothel, or a room I had dined in at an Aspen, Colorado restaurant many years earlier.

At the end of the dinner, I presented Jim with a scale replica of his Super Chipmunk complete with the 'Fang' emblem painted on the pilot's side of the cockpit (see photo below with Jim standing on the Chipmunk's wing). Needless to say, he was pleasantly surprised and delighted with that gift.

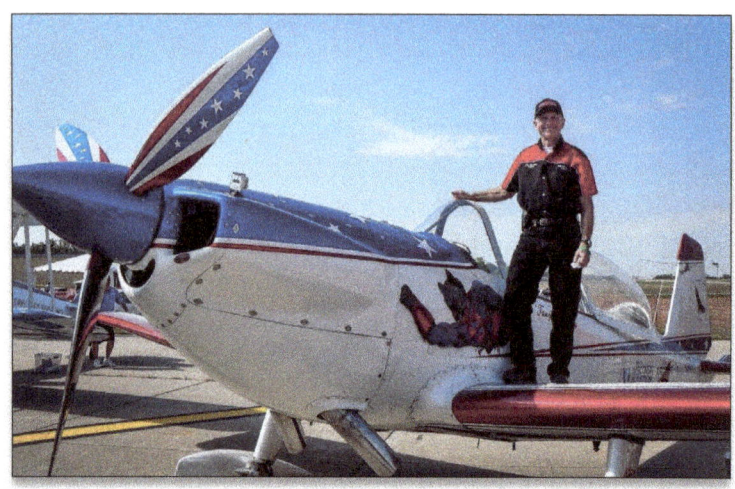

In 2013, my application to renew my NIH grant did not receive a fundable priority score, a situation that left me unable to support my laboratory activities going forward. I was going to resign my position as a Senior Investigator at the BRI, but I delayed that decision because there were some experimental 'loose ends' that I wanted to complete before I retired. Instead, I engineered a collaborative arrangement with the BloodCenter Diagnostics Laboratory to share the costs of investigating and developing a new assay that I had been working on.

In order to fund that project, I decided to sell 9390P and I placed ads in several places. After it had been on the market for several months, I received an offer from an army physician who was stationed in Germany at the time. I accepted a deposit and was preparing to close on its sale when I met with Jim for one of our usual lunch dates.

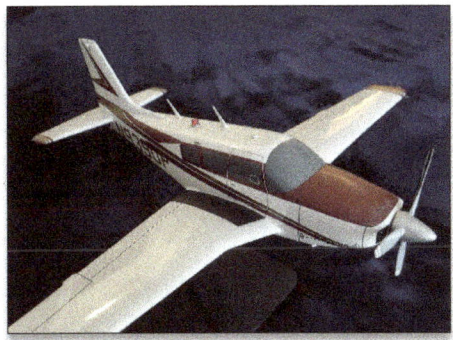

He had mentioned on several occasions that he wanted to buy 9390P for his retirement, but we never got much beyond a casual discussion of that subject. At lunch I explained to him that I had recently received a firm offer for the plane.

Jim quickly responded, "I still want to buy that plane."

"Jim," I said, "how much can you offer me for 9390P?" and I added, "because I want to use proceeds from the sale to fund an upcoming research project at the BloodCenter."

Jim was undeterred. He told me exactly how much he could pay for 9390P. That amount was lower than the offer already in hand, but it was close to the amount I would need for my research project.

I made an instant decision to accept his offer and we sealed the deal with a handshake. A few days later 9390P belonged to him, and I had contacted the army physician to return his deposit.

The same day that he took ownership of 9390P, Jim flew it from Timmerman Field to the Watertown airport where he kept his other airplanes. Before he left, I presented him with a replica of 9390P (*above*) to display alongside his replica of the Super Chipmunk.

During the next month Jim took me for some nostalgic 'right seat' rides in 9390P. (I could not fly left seat because Jim's insurance policy stipulated that only he could operate the aircraft as 'pilot-in-command'.) Despite that inconvenience, I enjoyed those flights immensely.

The Legend Grows

A few months later on March 23, 2014, Jim died in a night-time crash of his Super Chipmunk in mountainous terrain in the Cherokee National Forest in Tennessee while enroute to Smyrna, Florida for an airshow. It took several days to retrieve the wreckage and his body from the crash site.

Months later, The National Transportation Safety Board (NTSB) published the results of their investigation into the accident. On the evening of the crash, mountain tops in the area were reportedly obscured by clouds. Maroney had attempted to 'exit the weather' by flying beneath the cloud deck in a northerly heading when it impacted a mountain ridge one-hundred feet below its summit. The Chipmunk was not equipped with instrumentation that would have enabled him to safely enter or climb above the existing cloud layer.

Jim's remains were brought to Fargo, North Dakota, his hometown, for burial. Susan had the Super Chipmunk repaired and put on display in the Fargo Air Museum. Many of the Delta Airline pilots who had been under his command came to a memorial service that was held at the Watertown airport. Shirley and I were there.

Jim's airplanes, except for The Super Chipmunk, were on display and they included 'Little Toot' (*below left*), a single seat acrobatic biplane, an MS-X (*below right*) that Jim may have flown in 'pylon air races', and 9390P.

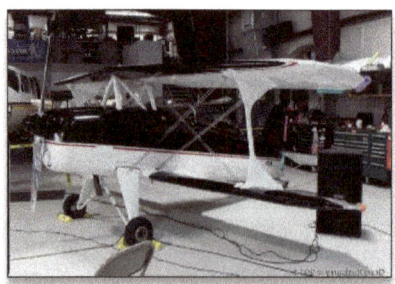 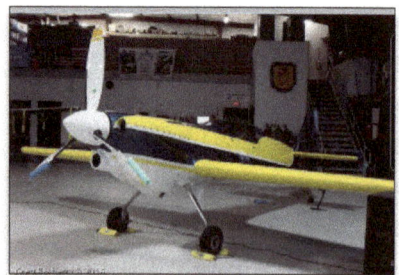

The memorial ceremony included a 'missing pilot' fly-by formation (*below*).

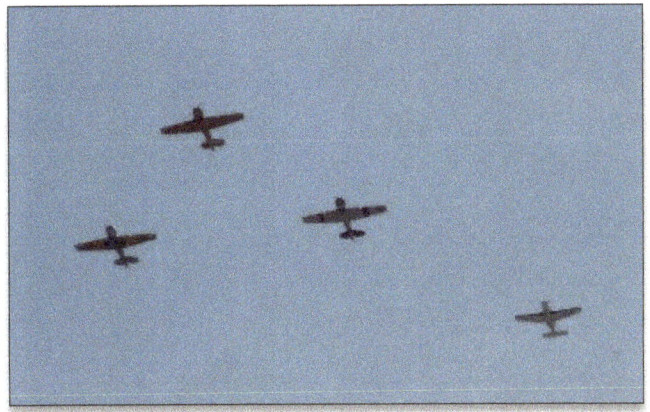

Susan Maroney was completely devastated by Jim's death. She returned to work at the BRI after grieving at home for several weeks. To date, although she soldiers on at the BRI she has not recovered from the loss of the love of her life. In recent years, meetings between us have been sad events for both of us because of the memories of Jim that we share.

Postscript

Susan was the heir to Jim's belongings and shortly after the Watertown memorial service had taken place, she put all of his airplanes on the market, including 9390P. I learned later that the army physician who had previously wanted to buy 9390P, had continued tracking its whereabouts. When he found out that it was again for sale, he contacted the Watertown airplane broker and bought 9390P. The plane now resides with him somewhere in Texas. The legend of Jim Maroney, the aviator, my friend, has now been written and hopefully will enable it to live on.

Michael Mosesson

Chapter 7

RESUSCITATION WITH A TWIST

Jim Maki, Bob Hudy, and I were enjoying a round of golf together at the Grant Park golf course on a windy afternoon in May 2019. We were about to tee off at the fifteenth hole when Hudy suddenly collapsed between the tee markers with his driver in hand. To say the least, that disrupted what should have been an uneventful day.

We were members of the Brown Deer Senior Men's Golf Club and were planning to play that day in a club-sponsored tournament at the Hidden Glen Golf Club in Cedarburg, but recent heavy downpours had inundated the course and the course manager decided that the course was too wet to allow motorized golf carts. Only golfers who carried their own clubs or used push carts would be allowed to play. None of us wanted to walk that course and we cancelled our reservation. Instead, we booked a round at the Grant Park golf course on the southside of Milwaukee, which was allowing motorized carts that day.

The weather was cool and windy, but fine for golf. Maki and I rode together in one cart and Hudy drove another. Everything went well until we arrived at the fifteenth tee. Hudy led the way and headed to the tee, with driver in hand. Jim Maki and I got out of our cart and retrieved our own drivers. As I turned toward the tee, I saw Bob lying spread eagled between the tee markers.

I dropped my club and ran to where he was lying. He was motionless and not breathing, his eyes were narrow slits with only the white sclera showing. I reached for his wrist and did not detect a pulse.

Hudy was on his back and well-positioned for Cardio-Pulmonary Resuscitation (CPR). I immediately began compressing his chest (sternum) with my hands positioned one on top of the other at about 70 to 75 compressions per minute. I asked Jim Maki to monitor Hudy's pulse.

After about two minutes of CPR Hudy suddenly took a few breaths and then again stopped breathing. I continued the chest compressions for what seemed like an eternity, but actually was only fifty to sixty seconds, when he resumed breathing irregularly. A short time later, he moved his lips and arms, made some sounds and gestures, and opened his eyes. I stopped the chest compressions, reached for his wrist and found that his pulse was rapid and regular! A minute or so later he attempted to sit up. I restrained him at first, but when he began to retch, I helped him sit up. The entire episode had lasted not more than five minutes.

Hudy remained seated on the ground for another minute or so while Jim Maki and I figured out what to do next. The 15th tee at Grant Park was located as far from the clubhouse as it could be, and we realized that we needed to get there as soon as possible.

Jim Maki was more agile and stronger than me, and he helped Bob to stand. He then led him to one of the carts and helped him climb aboard. Hudy remained dazed and speechless as we set out for the clubhouse with Maki and him in the lead and me following close behind. When we were about halfway to the clubhouse, Hudy began to retch again. That caused us to pause for a minute or two before resuming the ride to the clubhouse.

Once we arrived at the clubhouse our next problem was getting Hudy to a hospital. I suggested that we call 911 and wait for an ambulance to arrive, but Maki had a different idea. He estimated that since the nearest hospital, St Francis, was only ten minutes away by car, he suggested instead that it would be faster to drive him there in one of our cars. I agreed, we loaded Hudy into Jim's car, and off we went.

When we arrived at the St. Francis Emergency Room

entrance, I went inside to summon the aids to bring a gurney or a wheelchair. They brought a wheelchair and transported Hudy into the ER. By then he was fully awake though still incoherent and still retching. ER personnel then monitored his vital signs, administered IV fluids, monitored his EKG, and drew blood for testing.

After one hour they informed us that they did not have proper equipment for interrogating or adjusting his pacemaker, or for rendering advanced cardiac care.[16] Accordingly, they transferred him to Froedtert Hospital where he remained for two or three days before being discharged to home. Two weeks later Bob was planning his next golf round. Jokingly, I suggested that on our next round of golf we'd penalize him two strokes for 'delay-of-game', but of course I never did.

The Twist

About two years later (August 2021), in my search for a place to move after having sold my apartment at The Newport, I visited Newcastle Place, a senior residence in Mequon, Wisconsin. *Alicia Diedrich*, my host that day, was shepherding me around the facility and showing me amenities and features that I had not seen in previous visits. We stopped at The Snack Bar for lunch and soon after we had sat down, I said to her with some confidence, that at my age, I might become the oldest male resident in that community. Alicia responded with surprise and laughter as she gestured to someone else in the cafe, "….that man there is ninety-nine years old." She was pointing to *Jim Partleton*.

---

[16] Later interrogations of Hudy's pacemaker at Froedtert Hospital revealed that he'd had two episodes of ventricular tachycardia (VT), the first one at 1:29 PM and the second a few seconds later. Hudy's twitching that I observed during CPR might have been due to discharges from the defibrillator.

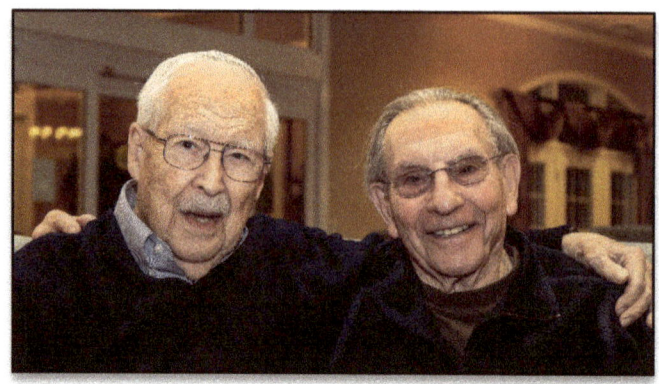

Using Alicia's response as an introduction, I promptly walked over to Partleton to engage him in conversation. He told me that he was still physically fit, still played golf, and still enjoying life there after having lived for eighteen years as a Newcastle resident. Meeting him was all I needed to make my decision and a few weeks later I moved to Newcastle Place.

During my first few weeks at Newcastle Place, I ran into Jim several times and each time we had a lengthy and pleasant conversation. During one of those encounters he told me that during a recent visit to his daughter's home in Shorewood, he had mentioned my name to her. To his surprise she told him she knew who I was and that two years earlier I had saved *Lynn Hudy's* husband Bob's life at the Grant Park Golf Course. To end our conversation that day, Partleton jokingly said that he was not sure whether or not to thank me for saving his son-in-law's life.[17]

Michael Mosesson

---

[17] Bob Hudy continued to play golf until a few months before his death in April 2023.

Chapter 8

SHIRLEY ANN (McDOWELL) MOSESSON
Love, Circumstance, Grief, Recovery

It is difficult to describe the sadness and emptiness I experienced shortly after Shirley, my wife of forty-seven years, died on May 14, 2015. The factors leading to my profound grief included the unbreachable gap that death had created, coupled with the belief that life had little more to offer. At my request, *Gil Church*, my long-time friend, trial lawyer, ordained minister, and Islamic scholar, conducted Shirley's memorial service. My hope was that his wisdom and counsel would afford me some relief, but they did not. I remember him looking at me to say, '*Grief is the other side of love*'. I did not grasp its meaning until years later while I was writing this chapter about Shirley Ann Mosesson.

Our story began in St. Louis in 1963 at Washington University School of Medicine. *Sol Sherry*, a renowned physician/scientist, Professor of Medicine, and head of *The Enzymology Section*, a *fibrinolysis* research group, had offered me an opportunity to complete medical residency training on the Barnes Hospital Ward Medical Service. My name had been brought to his attention by his associates, *Tony Fletcher* and *Norma Alkjaersig*, whom I had recently met at a hematology conference in Mexico where I presented some of the research that I had recently carried out at DBS. The subject of my presentation involved *fibrinolysis*, a subject that undoubtedly prompted their referring me to *Sol Sherry*. Prior to that offer I had considered going back to New York to complete residency training at Bellevue Hospital (NYU Medical School). I also considered returning to my alma mater, Downstate Medical Center, to begin a surgical residency with a former mentor, *Clarence Dennis*,

Chairman of The Department of Surgery, but the offer from Sol Sherry was irresistible and my next stop was St Louis.

During my stay in St. Louis, I completed my medical residency requirements and at the same time spent time as a research/clinical fellow in the Hematology section and in Sol Sherry's Enzymology Section. All of these activities were helpful for my development as a Physician/Scientist.

Personal experiences were equally good. I made many friends, went on numerous skiing expeditions to Colorado, played in too-high stakes poker games to my chagrin, enhanced my abilities as a pilot and earned new flight ratings. And of course, I met *Shirley Ann McDowell*.

Shirley was a charge nurse on one of Barnes Hospital's surgical services to which I had been summoned for a medical consultation on a patient requiring medical clearance before surgery. I was stricken by her good looks, grace and charm and almost immediately began to pursue her. It wasn't long before I fell in love with her. It was a bit longer before she reciprocated.

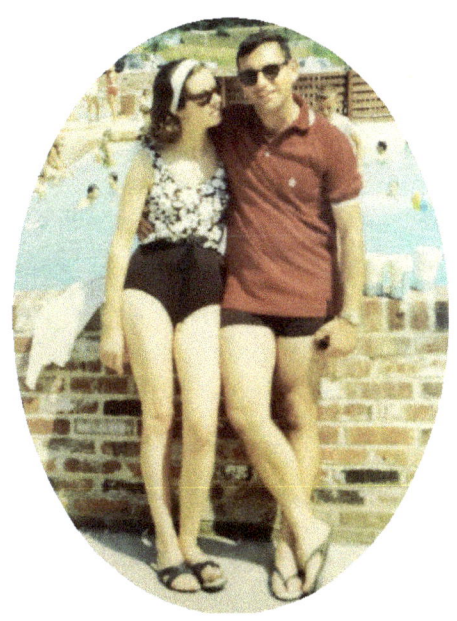

The courtship was not always smooth. One bump came at the beginning of our relationship. Shirley was raised in Princeton, Indiana, a small town where Jewish people were unknown and where antisemitism was baked into the local culture. She brought that attitude with her to St Louis. It took one or two earnest discussions to change that attitude, and after her epiphany, antisemitism was never again an important topic for discussion.

Even as our relationship developed, she remained in the thrall of a previous boyfriend, someone named *John Hatly*. Her episodic liaisons with him almost led to our breakup. During our second year together, without explanation, she cancelled our New Year's Eve date so she could spend time with Hatly. That experience had been unsettling, but nonetheless, two weeks later we had patched things up and were together once again.

Memories of the New Year's Eve experience fanned doubts in my mind about our long-range prospects and delayed further discussion of that subject for months, until a few weeks before my planned departure from St. Louis for a faculty appointment at my alma mater, SUNY Downstate.

In April that year, Shirley and I traveled to Effingham, Illinois, for the wedding of her best friend, *Marilynn Wolf,* to *Charles Anderson,* one of the surgical residents at Barnes Hospital. Shirley and I spent that night together. A few weeks later, shortly before I was to leave for New York, she informed me that she was pregnant. Following a brief discussion we both agreed that we were destined to be together. That July, shortly after we had moved to New York, we were married by a reform Rabbi (in deference to my mother's wish for a Jewish wedding). Our first home was in an apartment at 20 Cliff Street on Staten Island, a building almost in the shadow of the Verrazano Narrows Bridge. Our son, *Matthew Norman,* was born on January 1, 1968.

From that time forward, our lives blended into a loving, intimate, caring, and joyful affair. Two years later we welcomed *Marni Helene* and four years after that *Aimee Francine* came aboard. In the decades that followed, Shirley and I worked harmoniously in raising our children, guiding their education, planning their marriages, and sharing innumerable other pleasant experiences.

Among our shared experiences was a sabbatical year in Paris with the children. Three years later, we moved from Rockville Centre, New York, to Milwaukee, Wisconsin, where I became Vice Chairman of The Department of Internal Medicine and Director of the Winter Research Institute at Sinai Samaritan 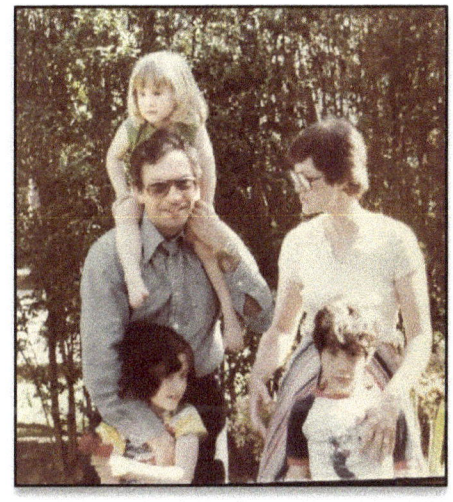 Hospital, a clinical teaching campus of The University of Wisconsin Medical School in Madison. I was successful in that position, and remained until 1999 when, for a multitude of reasons, I moved my research grants and activities to The Blood Research Institute (BRI) of The BloodCenter of Wisconsin.

In 1996, we brought my mother, *Esther*, from her life-long existence in Brooklyn, New York, to live at Chai Point, a Jewish-oriented retirement community in Milwaukee. Four years later, at the age of 94, she died from Legionnaire's disease that had been complicated by a thrombotic stroke. Shirley had grown very fond of her and was distraught at her passing. It seemed no coincidence that one week following Esther's death, Shirley suffered a stroke herself that left her with significant left-sided weakness. That disability and other emerging health issues served to strengthen the bond between us. I became her devoted and loving caregiver for the remainder of her life.

Shirley's Death

In 2013, after spending fourteen years as Senior Investigator at the BRI, I closed my laboratory and at the same time began exploring senior retirement communities in the Milwaukee area. After several months of searching, we decided on *St. Johns On The Lake*, a community near our apartment at The Newport.

Late in March 2015, one week after our return from a two-week vacation in Phoenix Arizona, we went for dinner at Kiku, a Japanese restaurant in downtown Milwaukee. Following our dinner, we left the restaurant in good spirits, returned to our apartment and went to bed at around 10 PM. I fell asleep with Shirley nestled in my arms.

I awakened the next morning at the same moment that she left the bed to go to the bathroom. When she didn't return within a minute, I sat up and turned in her direction. She looked startled and was leaning on the bathroom sink counter with her good right arm. I realized that something was seriously wrong, leaped out of bed and got to her side just as she began to collapse. I threw my arms around her, brought her back to the bed, and called 911 to summon an ambulance which arrived a short time later.

The ambulance attendants transported Shirley to a nearby hospital, Columbia St Mary's, and I followed close behind in our car.

Less than two hours after her admission to the hospital, the so-called 'clot buster' drug, tPA, was administered. The relatively short time delay between symptom onset and tPA administration made me unrealistically optimistic about reversing her symptoms. Although there was moderate improvement in her condition after tPA administration, my intital expectations did not materialize. By the second hospital day, although Shirley's slurred speech and swallowing difficulties had improved, her voice volume remained low, and the dense bilateral paresis had not changed.

A few days later, she began physical and occupational therapy and former medications, Plavix and mini-dose aspirin, were reinstituted. Another drug, Lamictal, which she had been taking for a recent mood disorder, was mistakenly dosed at three times her previous dose, a serious oversight that resulted in increased lethargy.

Several days after the dose of Lamictal had been adjusted, her lethargy diminished, and her swallowing and speaking disabilities improved. After she had spent three weeks at St Mary's, I arranged her transfer to the rehabilitation unit at St. John's On The Lake, the place we had chosen for our eventual retirement home.

The experience at the St John's rehabilitation unit was a nightmare for both of us, and it turned out to be a death sentence for Shirley. While she was there, I spent most days with her from mid-morning until after dinner. I was never comfortable about her well-being at that rehab unit, especially when I was not there to monitor what was going on.

I cannot recall a single day when the nursing or supportive care was satisfactory. Much of my dissatisfaction concerned the long delay that occurred whenever she signaled with her bedside buzzer for assistance or that she wanted to be taken to the restroom. Often, when she had been brought to the restroom, she was abandoned for extended periods and left sitting on the toilet seat. Similar long delays occurred when she signaled that she wanted her position adjusted or needed other assistance such as help in getting dressed, brushing her teeth or combing her hair. There were other serious problems such as leaving her to eat on her own without monitoring or assistance during mealtimes when I wasn't there to help her.

I complained bitterly and loudly almost every day to nursing staff, floor administrators, and even to the St John's president. I routinely experienced vacuous assurances of changes that were never implemented.

Early one May morning, I was awakened at home by a call from a floor nurse at St John's who told me that Shirley had aspirated some food at breakfast time and was having difficulty breathing. No one had been with her when the incident occurred, and she was uncertain how long she had been in distress. I demanded that she be taken to a hospital immediately, and a short time later, she was transferred by ambulance to Sinai Samaritan Hospital.

I arrived at the hospital shortly afterward and hurried to her room. She was on nasal oxygen, her blood oxygen saturation level was within normal limits, and she was able to hold a conversation. Her ability to cough was impaired and therefore she was could not bring up any aspirated material. Tracheal suctioning was attempted on several occasions with limited success.

The following week a chest X-ray showed that she had developed pneumonitis and that fluid had accumulated in her lungs. Increased amounts of nasal oxygen were required to maintain normal blood oxygen saturation. Day by day she grew weaker and less able to cough or bring up material from her lungs. Because of difficulty in swallowing, a radiological investigation of her swallowing ability was performed. Shortly after completing that study and had returned to her room she again aspirated some fluid. Following that incident, she was not able to maintain a safe blood oxygen level. She refused airway suctioning, even though she realized that it was the only procedure that might have helped her.

90

I listened to Shirley in disbelief as she whispered to me that she was exhausted and wanted to give up. A short time later, one of her physicians pulled me aside to tell me that there was nothing more that could be done for her. I was presented with a 'Hobson's choice'—transfer her to a hospice for terminal care or provide hospice care at the hospital. I chose the latter.

Shirley and I were left alone in the room. Shirley's oxygen mask was removed, and an intravenous morphine drip was started to relieve her respiratory discomfort. I climbed into her bed and held her in my arms. The room was silent, and her eyes were closed. I whispered to her that I loved her. Her last words were, "I love you, too". A few minutes or perhaps hours later, I cannot recall, she stopped breathing.

The Road to Recovery

I had lost my life partner, and the grief that followed was unrelenting. I was inconsolable, directionless, and uncomfortably alone in my apartment, or when I could not bear being by myself, I would drive to my daughter Aimee's home in Chicago to spend a day or two with her before returning to Milwaukee.

After three months had passed, with prodding from my friends, I signed up with a University of Wisconsin sponsored organization named OSHER that offered educational and other experiences to seniors. I enrolled in a French literature discussion class that provided the opportunity to refresh and maintain the fluency in French that I had developed during our stay in Paris.

Another aspect of my recovery plan included an online subscription to *Match.com.* I contacted several women through that website, met a few for coffee, lunch, or dinner. None of these meetings panned out and after a few months I dropped the subscription and returned to full-time grieving.

Recovery and Beyond

For the first few weeks after Shirley's death, Aimee handled the mail and other correspondence that arrived at our home. That included responding on my behalf to all the condolence cards that arrived. One of those cards was sent by *Libby Temkin*, but I was unaware of it for many months.

The following April, still unaware of having received her condolence card, I came across a Facebook posting by Libby Temkin, a photo of her with her family at a Brewer's baseball game. I had not seen her since her husband Sher's memorial service five years earlier. I wrote a comment on her page, reintroduced myself, and asked whether she might be interested in meeting me for coffee. A few days later she replied in the affirmative.

Our first meeting took place a few weeks later at Café Hollander on Downer Avenue. I was surprised when she told me that she knew about Shirley's passing and that she had sent a condolence card. She also told me that she was in a 'committed relationship' with a man from St. Louis named *Les Nackman*. Despite this disclosure, we continued meeting for coffee and often for dinner. The dinner conversations were pleasant and sometimes involved hand-holding and other affectionate exchanges.

One evening, as I prepared to drop her off at her home after a dinner date, she took hold of my tie, pulled me into her house and then to her bedroom, an experience that I soon became accustomed to.

In the weeks that followed my fondness for Libby increased, and judging from her behavior, so did hers for me. My grieving had dissipated, and my life was taking a new shape. By October, Libby ended her 'committed relationship' with Nackman, and turned her attention entirely to me.

That November, she invited me to spend the winter with

her at her Florida home in Boca Raton, and I accepted. The following spring, after another enjoyable winter together, we returned to Milwaukee and resumed our romance at her home in Mequon. The winter, 'snowbird'/spring, Milwaukee migrations continued for four years. During the four years we were together in unwedded bliss, I rarely stayed at my apartment, and instead spent most days and nights at her place. I was happy to leave my memories of Shirley at The Newport.

At the beginning of our fifth year together, Libby put her Florida home on the market and by October she had closed on the sale. Our relationship had been so solid for so long that I naïvely assumed that we would be together for the long term. With those thoughts uppermost in my mind, I put my apartment on the market, a decision that she seemed to welcome at first.

By March, I had sold my apartment and began disposing of my furniture and other belongings. These items included a baby grand piano that had been in my possession for more than seventy years. Among the few items I brought with me to Mequon were a few cartons containing CDs, photo albums, porcelain dishes, silverware, clothing, paintings, and other artefacts. I also brought two office chairs, one of which was intended for Libby's use. That was it!

Libby's behavior and attitude changed during the transition. She seemed angered at the boxes and other items that I had brought with me. At first, I ignored this, but during the next few weeks her discontent became more apparent and sometimes hostile.

We had been together for more than four years, happily I thought, but that was no longer true. We communicated more infrequently, and during the last few weeks at her home I slept alone in another part of the house. That October, I moved to Newcastle Place.

It would be an understatement to say that I was angry and confused about how the relationship had deteriorated. About a year later, after I had moved to Newcastle Place, I received a letter from Libby's nephew, *Larry Temkin*, who wrote to me about her discontent. He explained that the reason for Libby's changed attitude was her fear of ever again becoming a caregiver for someone, as had occurred with Sher, her husband. That letter helped me find closure (see Chapter 10).

I still care about Libby Temkin, but no longer am I troubled by the situation that evolved. I'm relieved that this episode in my life has passed and that I have emerged intact on the other side of it. I will always be grateful to Libby for having been the instrument for my recovery from grief over Shirley Ann (McDowell) Mosesson.

One Last Item

There remained one loose end for me to address before I could achieve the closure I needed. Shirley's ashes had been in my possession for more than seven years. During that period, I tried several times, unsuccessfully, to find a suitable place for her remains. I had discussed that with my children on numerous occasions, but inertia prevailed.

That situation changed a few months after I had relocated to Newcastle Place. My apartment on the second floor of the North Building had a balcony with an expansive view of the surrounding woods and ponds. For several weeks I explored those woods and wandered through many of the trails. Finally, I found a suitable place for Shirley's remains, one that I could view from the balcony.

In January I took several pictures of the surrounding woods, most of them at sunrise. With the photos in hand, I approached my friend, fellow golfer, and artist, *Jim Maki*, and commissioned him to render a painting of that view. A few weeks later he presented me with the completed painting (*below*). It now resides on a wall in my apartment near the balcony. It is both a tribute to Shirley's memory and a guidepost to her resting

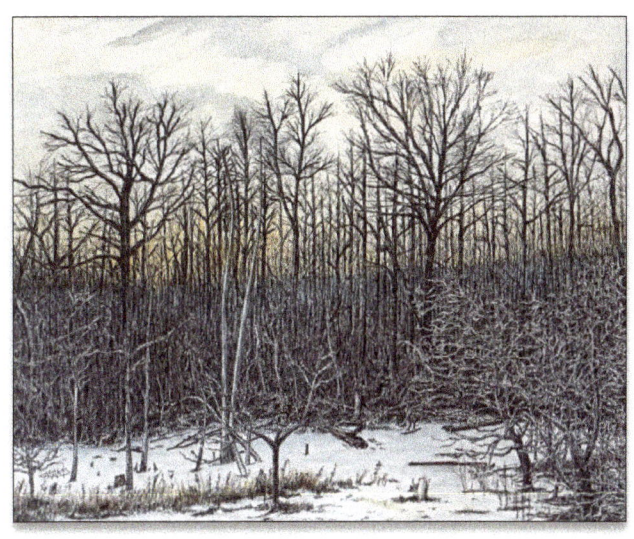

Jim Maki's painting of the view from the balcony, a site that contained a snow-covered pond at the time. Shirley's remains are located in the woods just to the right of the pond.

place. Shortly after the painting had been completed, I organized a memorial celebration for Shirley that would be shared with my children, their families, and Shirley's niece and nephew, Joyce and Mark McDowell[18]. On July 31, 2022, they came to share their thoughts and memories. The site where each one of us deposited some of her ashes is marked by a plaque mounted on a nearby tree.

Michael Mosesson

---

[18] Mark was not able to be at the July 31st celebration, but a few months later he and his wife, Joyce, came to Newcastle Place to visit Shirley's gravesite and close the circle.

Chapter 9

'GRANDPA IS MY DADDY'

In July 1975, Shirley and I travelled to Paris, France to attend a scientific conference. After eight years of marriage our family had expanded by three: Matt (1968), Marni (1969), and Aimee (1974). While we were away, my parents, *Benjamin* and *Esther Mosesson*, cared for them at our home in Rockville Centre.

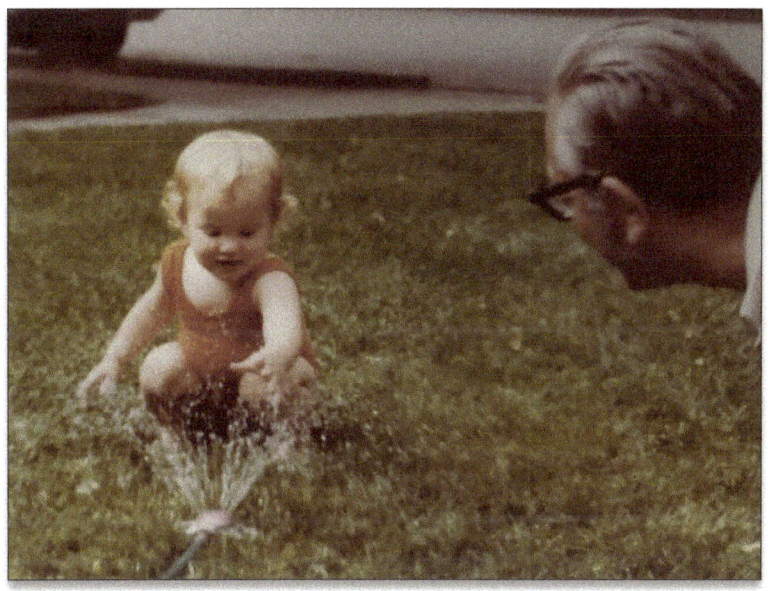

Aimee and my dad, Benjamin, at our home in Rockville Centre

We lodged at Hotel de Nice on Boulevard Raspail, a setting conducive to 'romantic encounters'. Later that summer, a few weeks after we had returned from France, Shirley informed me that she was pregnant once again. I was delighted at that news and quite certain that the pregnancy had been launched on Boulevard Raspail. Shirley did not share that enthusiasm and instead, she became quite dour. The outcomes from that announcement are the basis for this story/fantasy.

The Beginning of Our Story

Shirley Ann McDowell and I first met in St. Louis, Missouri, while I was a medical resident at Barnes Hospital in St Louis. One evening, I responded to a request from the surgical service for a medical consultation on one of their patients. Shirley was the charge nurse on that ward. After attending to the consultation request, I then turned my attention to that lovely and charming nurse. That encounter marked the beginning of a courtship that lasted for more than three years until just weeks before I was scheduled to leave for a new position at SUNY Downstate Medical Center in Brooklyn, New York when I finally proposed marriage to her, and she accepted.

We were married on July 23, 1967, in Queens by a Jewish 'reform' rabbi (no other self-respecting Rabbi would have agreed to create a union between a goy and a Jew) and began our lives together in an apartment building on Cliff Street in Staten Island that was located in the shadow of the Verrazzano Narrows suspension bridge connecting Staten Island to Brooklyn. Matthew was born 'prematurely' the following January and Marni was born 19 months later. A few months after that, I began to lobby for a third child. Shirley was not the least bit enthusiastic about my lobbying, and after a few weighty conversations we dropped the subject from our discussion agenda.

Four years later, in the fall of 1973, Shirley became pregnant once again. She was not overjoyed at the prospect of having another child, but after considerable discussion and cajoling, her reticence receded. On May 25, 1974, we welcomed *Aimee Francine* to the family. (*Aimee* is the American English version of the French word for love, *aimé*.)

Our Fourth Child

A few months prior to Aimee's birth, we moved from Staten Island, the 'fifth borough', to a four-bedroom house on Arizona Avenue in Rockville Centre, Long Island. About one year later, when Aimee was 14 months of age, we left our children in the care of my parents and set out for the aforementioned visit to France. A few weeks after our return, Shirley announced that she was pregnant again.

As before, I was pleased at the idea of having another child, but Shirley was not. She was firm in her insistence that she did not want to carry that pregnancy. I tried to convince her that 'number four' would be another '*love child*' and a welcomed addition to our family, but she remained implacably negative despite all my cajoling and pleading.

One morning late in September, without informing me about her intention, she left home and drove to Downstate Medical Center for an appointment with her obstetrician, *George Solish*, who was a faculty colleague of mine. George performed the abortion that same day.

After learning what had occurred, I was angry and disappointed, and I told her so. In the weeks that followed, we had several heated discussions. Although the choice to end the pregnancy was hers to make, I nevertheless argued vehemently that her action had been hurtful to all of us. Toward the end of these arguments, she became remorseful and mindful of the gravity of her fateful decision.

During one confrontation, I went so far as to suggest that we end our marriage, but she declined that option. I soon abandoned that idea when I realized that my love for her had not diminished, and that divorce could not resolve or reverse what had happened.

Shirley had no way of knowing that the abortion occurred a few weeks before my father, Benjamin David Mosesson, passed away from a heart attack. His death made her act even more onerous for me, since the birth of that child would have presented a timely opportunity to honor my father's memory.

Moving On

My anger gradually faded, and we settled into a more normal non-argumentative existence. I began developing plans for a sabbatical leave in France at Hôpital Beaujon in Clichy, France, a visit that would be sponsored by my friend and colleague, *Doris Ménaché*. I enrolled in Alliance Française and two years later, in July 1977, we sailed on the QE II to Le Havre, France to begin the adventure.

That year in France was a rewarding cultural and educational experience for everyone, and it presented an opportunity for us to further heal the rift that had existed for several years. I also achieved my scientific goal of successfully investigating a family from Paris with a congenital abnormality of plasma fibrinogen, a *dysfibrinogenemia*, that came to be known as '*Fibrinogen Paris I*'. That abnormality had been discovered by *Doris Ménaché* and was the second such dysfibrinogen to have been described.

The following year, with the investigation of Fibrinogen Paris-I under my belt, we returned to New York and resumed our former lives. That situation lasted for three years until I uprooted everyone again to accept an offer to join the faculty of the University of Wisconsin Medical School and develop a Research Division at Sinai Samaritan Medical Center in Milwaukee, Wisconsin. In July 1981, we moved to 2730 Menlo Boulevard in Shorewood.

Relocating to Wisconsin was life changing for everyone. For our children it meant adjusting to a new home, new schools, new friends and new relationships. For Shirley, it was a challenging adventure to which she responded enthusiastically. For me it involved all of the above plus an unprecedented

100

opportunity to enlarge and further develop my career as a scientist, teacher, and clinician.

Over the next few years, our family grew closer and more tightly knit, including the relationship between Shirley and me. The academic and research pursuits that had prompted the move far exceeded my expectations and memories of our lost child faded even further from my thoughts.

After graduating from Shorewood High School, *Matthew* enrolled at Purdue University and graduated four years later having majored in aeronautical engineering. A few years later, he married *Amber Jost* and they settled down in nearby Whitefish Bay. During the first years of their marriage Amber gave birth to *Harper* and *Arden*. Unfortunately, their marriage ended a few years later in an acrimonious and contentious divorce whose consequences still reverberate for all of us.

Marni graduated with a BA degree from Alverno College with a major in education. She married *Bill Kambol* and they had two children while together *Emma Grace* and *Luca*. After living for several years in Illinois, they moved to St Louis, Missouri, where Bill took a position at the Nestle Corporation, and Marni became a reading specialist in the St. Louis public school system. Their marriage also ended in divorce.

The Rest of The Story[19]

Aimee graduated with a BA degree from Miami of Ohio University in 1997. Two years later, she earned a master's degree in architecture at the UW Milwaukee School of Architecture, and then joined *Perkins and Will* to begin her architectural career.

In 2004, Aimee married *Christian Eckmann*, her longtime boyfriend from Miami of Ohio days. Christian became a chef who honed his culinary skills with an internship in San Sebastian, Spain. They settled in Chicago where Christian became an executive chef and corporate partner with 'Let Us Entertain You'. He managed several of their Chicago restaurants. He now owns and manages his own restaurant called *Asador Bastian*, an upscale chop house with a Spanish bent.

During the first few years of their marriage, Aimee had several spontaneous miscarriages. One of them occurred when we were together on a ski vacation at our condo in Dillon, Colorado. After so many unsuccessful tries, she must have wondered whether she would be able to carry a pregnancy to term. Happily, on July 12, 2012, she gave birth to a boy who they named *Sebastian*, a name based on Christian's San Sebastian experience.

---

[19] This subtitle paraphrases what *William Harvey*, the late radio broadcaster and inveterate storyteller, usually said when he segued to the end of a story, "*...and now for the rest of the story*".

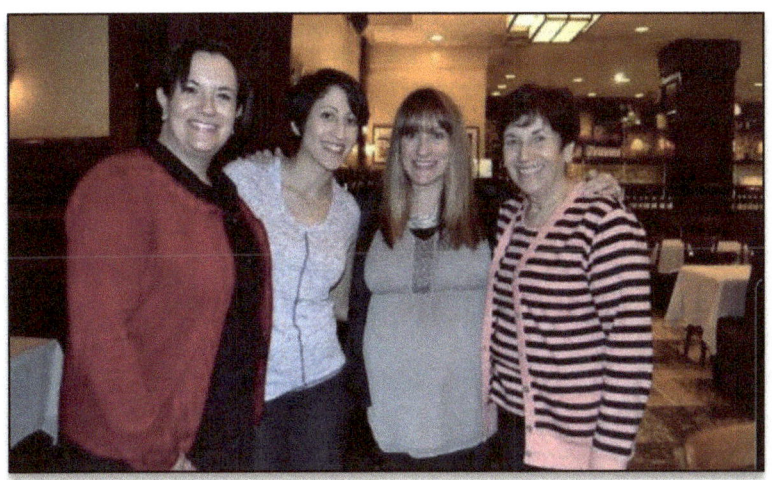

Marni, Beth Dembrow, Aimee, and my sister Judith Dembrow at the baby shower for Sebastian Bennjamin Anthony Eckmann.

I was delighted at the news of Sebastian's birth, and even more so when I learned that his second given name was *Benjamin* in honor of my father. He was also given a third name, *Anthony* in honor of Christian's grandfather.

We were all unprepared for the accident that occurred to Aimee when Sebastian was 15 months old. While descending a flight of stairs leading to her basement, Aimee, then 39 years of age, tripped and fell to the bottom of the stairwell. She suffered deep and painful bruising but fortunately there were no broken bones or other serious consequences, or so we thought.

A few days later after the fall, while she was recovering from the fall, she experienced the sudden onset of facial weakness and slurred speech, symptoms of a '*transient ischemic attack*' (TIA). That alarming and unforeseen event resulted in immediate hospitalization. Aimee telephoned to alert us, and we immediately drove from Milwaukee to the Northwestern University hospital in Chicago where she had been hospitalized. Fortunately, the TIA symptoms subsided within a few days, and she made an uneventful recovery.

There was no cogent explanation for why such a serious neurological event had occurred at such a young age to someone who previously had been in excellent health, and that led to a diagnostic search for a cause. In the days following the TIA, blood tests revealed an elevated blood level of lipoprotein A [LP(a)]. Elevated levels of this lipoprotein are hereditary in nature, and often are associated with the occurrence of thrombotic vascular events such as TIAs and strokes.

When I learned of Aimee's elevated LP(a) level I remembered that Shirley had previously experienced several TIAs prior to her thrombotic stroke in 2000, a stroke that left her with left-sided paresis. (Fifteen years later, she would have a second thrombotic stroke that eventually resulted in her death from aspiration pneumonia (chapter 8).) I also was aware that the McDowell family history included several close relatives who had suffered strokes, and that Aimee's own brother Matthew had recently suffered a minor thrombotic stroke at the age of forty. A short time later we learned that Shirley's blood LP(a) level was even higher than Aimee's, clearly implicating the hereditary nature of these thrombotic events. In Aimee's case, the TIA was probably induced by the extensive tissue damage she suffered when she fell down the stairs.[20]

---

[20] There is an association between elevated blood levels of LP(a) and the occurrence of TIAs, thrombotic strokes, and spontaneous miscarriages. The lipoprotein LP(a) binds to blood clots at sites that result in increased resistance of the clot to *fibrinolysis* [A biological process that leads to dissolution (lysis) of formed blood clots.]. High blood levels of LP(a) undoubtedly result in greater LP(a) binding to clots and increased resistance to fibrinolysis.

Undissolved blood clots can obstruct the flow of blood, an event that results in anoxic damage to the tissues and organs supplied by that blood vessel. When clot obstruction involves vessels supplying brain tissue, TIAs or thrombotic strokes occur. When obstruction involves placental blood vessels, miscarriages can result.

With this new information in hand, we turned to a physician (*Dr. Stone*) with experience in managing subjects with elevated LP(a) levels. Given Aimee's history of having had several miscarriages and, more recently, a TIA, plus the hypercoagulable state that inevitably accompanies pregnancy, he advised her to avoid another pregnancy. He also prescribed a 'statin' in order to *'passivate'* the endothelial lining of her blood vessels.

A few weeks after Shirley's death, *Jean Collins* invited me to join *The Miracles Group*. It was comprised of six people who met regularly to read aloud, discuss, and dissect the contents of a quasi-biblical book entitled '*A Course in Miracles*'. This book had its origins in the 1970's, mainly through the writings of a psychologist at Columbia University who had 'channeled' the verses over the course of several years, reportedly without knowledge of the origins or the source of what she transcribed. Her writings were eventually typeset and published in several languages. Its biblical-like character and messages spawned societies worldwide that were focused on analyzing its spiritual, ethical, and quasi-religious messages. Hence, our Miracles group.

The sessions usually began with a clockwise reading of passages, followed by lengthy and animated discussions of the textual meanings and interpretations. The meetings always ended in a joined-hands circle in silent contemplation.

It was at these meetings that I explored aspects of spirituality that touched on reincarnation and paranormal phenomena. Some of our meetings included anecdotes about human clairvoyance[21] and recollections of previous past lives.

One of these occurred one evening at dinner with Jean Collins, the coordinator and *de facto* leader of the group. The conversation started out with casual conversation but halfway through the meal, for no apparent reason, I spontaneously blurted out, "Jean, have you ever been beheaded?"

Without hesitating she calmly replied, "Yes I have."

She did not seem surprised by the question, and she immediately added a detailed account of her previous existence. I was incredulous but I could not dismiss that forthright response from my thoughts. And those memories remain with me.

---

[21] One clairvoyant about whom I learned was *Edgar Cayce* who was known as the 'Sleeping Prophet'. In his later years he founded 'The Association for Research and Enlightenment'. I read the book commemorating his life and describing his clairvoyant experiences.

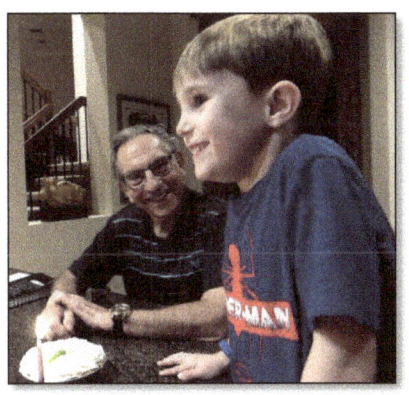

"Grandpa Is My Daddy"

During the months following Shirley's death, it was difficult for me to stay alone in my apartment, and I spent many weekends that summer and fall at Aimee's home. Sebastian was by then three years old and changing rapidly, especially concerning his speech and diction.

During one of those visits, while Sebastian and I were playing together, he turned to me and said, "*Grandpa is my daddy.*" And on my next visit he said the very same thing, "*Grandpa is my daddy.*"

I began to wonder, and I continue to wonder even now, whether there might be a *spiritual* interpretation to what Sebastian said. Could the spirit of the child which had years before resided in Shirley's womb, now reside with Sebastian? That answer will always be elusive, nebulous, and unknowable.

Whatever the truth of this fantasy may be, the thoughts do not go away. My love for Sebastian does not change, nor does my relationship with him as his grandfather. The *'Grandpa is my daddy'* episodes will remain with me for the remainder of my life and wherever my spirit goes next.

Michael Mosesson

Chapter 10

LIFE WITH THE TEMKIN TRIBE (1981-2022)
Sherwood and Libby Temkin

In July 1981, I resigned my position at SUNY Downstate Medical Center with the intent of joining The University of Wisconsin Medical School (Madison) faculty at Sinai Samaritan Medical Center (SSMC) which was home to 'The Milwaukee Clinical Campus' a clinical teaching site for the medical school. The most important reason for moving to Wisconsin was to become director of the newly established Research Division that was located near the hospital complex in a newly renovated four story 20,000 ft² building, *'The Winter Research Institute'*.

Shortly after arriving in Milwaukee with my family, I met *Libby (nee: Libby Lindenberg) and Sherwood (Sher) Temkin*. Their daughter, *Robyn*, had recently died from metastatic melanoma at the age of 22. To honor her memory and mitigate their grief, they founded the Robyn Temkin Memorial Fund. As the director of the Research Division, I was asked to help them achieve their goals and I accepted. During the next few years, I organized lecture-dinners, luncheons, lectureships, visiting professorships, and skin-screening clinics. I also used their fund to award research grants-in-aid that were focused on cancer-related projects.

Libby, always personable and charming, participated actively in these initiatives, as did Sher to a lesser extent. We became friends and eventually added a social component to the friendship that included a few dinner parties at our home in Shorewood.

After ten years of Temkin fund related activities, I asked Libby to become the 'lay' member of the Animal Care Committee at The Winter Research Institute. She accepted my invitation and served on the committee for more than five years.

In the mid 1990's she resigned that position because she and Sher were becoming seasonal 'snowbirds. Following that change, I lost contact with them for the next fifteen years.

In February 2011, *Richard Taylor*, Libby's son-in-law, with whom I sometimes played tennis at our athletic club, Le Club, notified me that Sher Temkin had died. He also informed me about the memorial service to be held in Sher's honor. I attended that service and spoke briefly with Libby to convey my condolences. After that brief encounter, I did not see or hear from her again until another five years had passed.

2015-2016

In March 2015, *Shirley Mosesson* suffered her second major stroke, and after a rocky course, she passed away that May. Her death launched a prolonged period of grieving, depression, and self-pity for me, as chronicled in chapter 8.

In May 2016, while I was surfing on Facebook, I came across Facebook post showing Libby at a Brewer's baseball game with members of her family. I sent a comment to her asking whether she might be interested in getting together with me for coffee. A few days later she replied that she was out of town but would contact me after her return to Milwaukee. A few days later we met at Café Hollander on Downer Avenue. During our lunch conversation, she told me that she had been in a 'committed   relationship' with a man from St Louis named *Les Nackman.*

Despite that entanglement I asked her to meet me again, and we did so in the weeks that followed. Most often we would meet for coffee, but sometimes for dinner. Since her relationship with Les Nackman was well known to her Milwaukee friends, she insisted that we meet at places where we would be unlikely to encounter any of them. That plan worked until it didn't.

One evening we ran into her friends, *Neville* and *Adrienne*

Sender, at Tess's, a neighborhood restaurant. Neville, an obstetrician, was also known to me from Sinai Samaritan days. With 'the-cat-now-out-of-the-bag', Libby next invited me to join her and some of her friends while they were lunching at Elsa's restaurant. When I showed up, she pretended that my presence had been a chance encounter, but I doubt that anyone was taken in by that antic.

After that, our relationship advanced rapidly. One evening at dinner, she surprised me with, *"Michael, you take my breath away."* She also said that years earlier she had developed a 'crush' on me. That same June evening, while I was dropping her off at her home, she took hold of my tie while we were standing in the driveway and with a mischievous smile she led me into the house, then into her bedroom where we disrobed and made love for the first time. That was an unexpected but pleasant experience that soon became a regular event. When her birthday rolled around that August, I gave her a watch engraved on the back with *'June 16, 2016'*, a date that recalled that first evening.

During our rapidly developing romance, Libby at first continued to make weekend trips to St. Louis to visit Nackman, but that October, she decided to modify the 'committed' part of their relationship. She told me that their relationship had been in decline for some time, and our recent liaison had served to hasten her decision.

A few days later their relationship ended abruptly at Lambert Field in St Louis just as she was about to board her flight to Milwaukee. Libby told Nackman that she had been dating someone in Milwaukee and asked him whether he would accept an additional component to their arrangement. Nackman was infuriated. He told her that he was aware that she had been dating someone else and then stormed out of the terminal, abruptly ending their relationship. I humorously characterized that event as having been *'Nackmanned'*. I could not imagine at that time that I would also be 'Nackmanned' a few years later.

Shortly after the breakup with Nackman, I began staying most nights with her at her home. Libby responded to that with enthusiasm and encouragement, and a few weeks later we officially announced our 'affair' at a brunch with her daughter, *Kim Taylor*, and Kim's husband, *Richard*. I was certain that Kim already knew about our situation because they didn't kept secrets from each other for very long. A short time later, I began to introduce her to my friends and close associates.

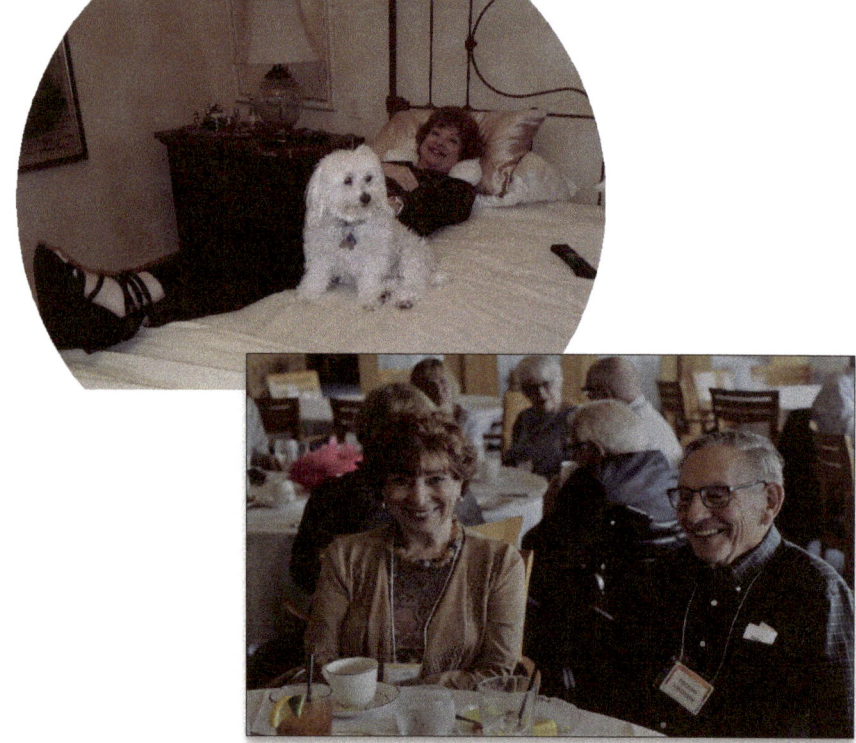

A Sinai Samaritan Staff Reunion, October 2016

Early in the relationship, Libby would sometimes say that she would be happy living alone. At first, that statement had little impact on me because my vision had been obscured by the fog of the love affair. We also discussed the possibility of marriage, but neither of us favored an arrangement that would certainly complicate our lives without improving it in any meaningful way, and the subject ceased to be a topic of conversation. Nevertheless, shortly after we began living together full time Libby gifted me a silver wedding band (*right*). It was her way, or so I thought, of underwriting our long-term relationship. I wore the ring from that time forward to indicate my own endorsement of the situation.

That first November, she invited me to spend the winter with her at her Florida home at The Boca Grove Country Club, and I accepted with enthusiasm. We did many things together that included frequent dinners at the Boca Grove Clubhouse or at outside restaurants, evenings at the Wick Theater and other entertainment venues, and weekend trips to places like The Kennedy Space Center. We bought a golf cart (*below*) for motoring around the country club grounds or for whenever I played golf ('Michael' was inscribed on one side-panel and 'Libby' on the other). In just a few months I had transitioned from a life of grieving and depression to one filled with love and happiness, one that would last for nearly five years.

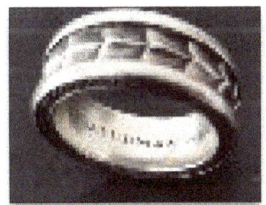

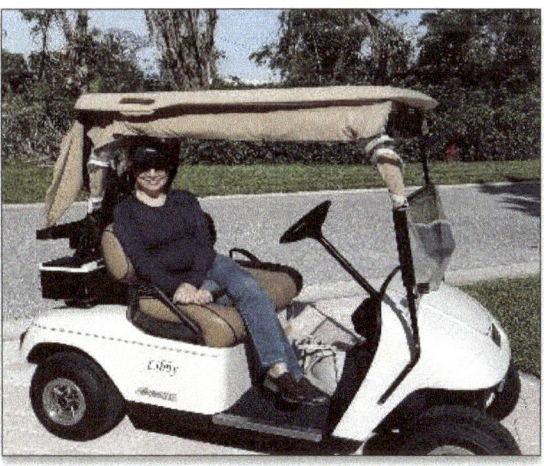

During our first three years together, we attended several Temkin family gatherings-I was delighted to have been invited

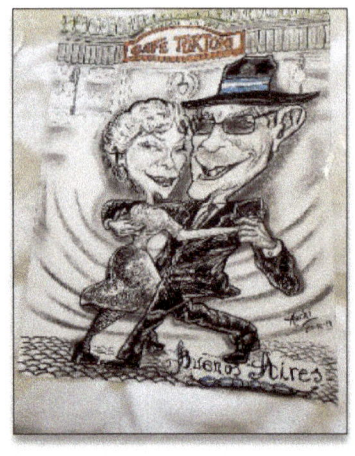

and have the opportunity to interact with so many of its members. I began to believe that I was an accepted member of the Temkin tribe.

In December of 2019, Libby organized a trip to Chile to visit her son, *Todd*, and his family where he had been living for more than twenty-five years. We were accompanied by her daughter, *Kim*, husband *Richard*, and their children *Ben and Olivia*. The visit was eventful and enjoyable from start to finish and included spending several days at Todd's ranch in Futaleufú, Patagonia. On the way back to Wisconsin, Libby and I spent some time in Buenos Aires *(above left)*.

A short time after our return from that trip, the COVID pandemic arrived in the United States (January 2020) with all its attendant restrictions and caveats about avoiding movies, restaurants, shows, plays or other public gatherings. Although these activities had been curtailed, we both enjoyed being 'cooped up' together at home.

That May, Libby and I planned to return to Wisconsin for the summer months, but since we were concerned about traveling in a commercial airliner during the COVID epidemic, we chartered an Embraer 300 jet to bring us and Alfie back to Milwaukee.

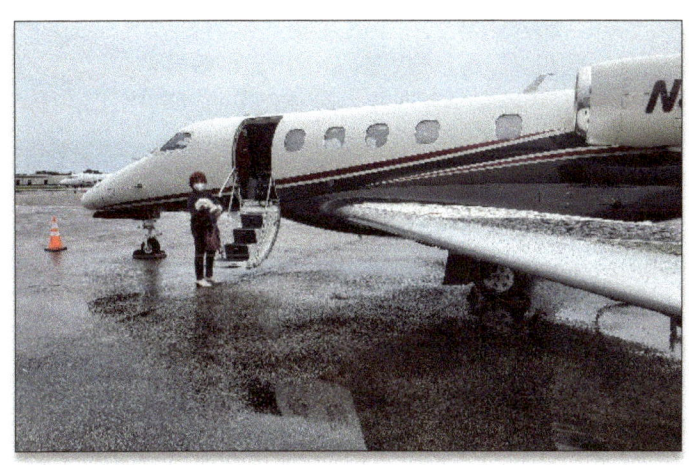

Selma Duckler and Fibrinogen Memoirs

Libby's sister, *Selma Duckler*, visited us several times from her home in Portland, Oregon, either in Wisconsin or in Florida. As told to me by Libby, both sisters had grown up in a stressful, sometimes abusive, family environment in La Cross, Wisconsin. But Selma's negative experiences, largely because she was the older sibling, were more stressful for her. They led to a near lifetime of psychiatric treatments and psychoanalysis. These were so important for her well-being that she maintained a close relationship with psychiatric societies and some former therapists, one of whom was *Arnold Richards*. On one of her visits to Florida, she arranged a dinner meeting that included Arnold Richards and his wife Arlene.

On the evening of that dinner, we arrived at the restaurant, Paradiso, several minutes before the Richards. The surname 'Richards' rang no bells for me, but the moment Arnold Richards entered the restaurant and came into view I remembered him as *Arnie Gorodowski*, a former classmate from Erasmus Hall High School in Brooklyn and from medical school at SUNY Downstate Medical Center. I shouted *"Arnie Gorodowski!"* and he soon responded, *"Michael Mosesson!"* The

115

dinner conversation that evening was replete with recollections and reactivation of our former friendship.

We met the Richards several more times during the next two years. One of our last meetings was for lunch, just weeks before Libby and I had planned on returning to Wisconsin. During that luncheon, Arnie revealed that in addition to having a successful career as a psychoanalyst, he had founded a publishing company called *IPBooks*. That revelation prompted a discussion about a manuscript I had been working on sporadically for more than ten years. At the time of our luncheon, I had completed an untitled draft, and I asked him to read it and let me know whether it might be worth publishing. He agreed to do so.

A few days later, along with some constructive comments and suggestions, he told me that IPBooks would be willing to publish my book. With that as encouragement, I quickly updated and revised the manuscript, and within a few weeks I had completed that task. I chose '*Fibrinogen Memoirs*' for the title and '*Journeys of a Clot Doctor*' for the subtitle. The book was published in 2020. For an encore I wrote *Fibrinogen Memoirs 2,* which was published by IPBooks in 2022.

Don't Say N***** If You Are Not Black

On May 10, 2020, Libby and I arrived at Milwaukee's Mitchell Field in the Embraer 300 jet that we had chartered. Libby's granddaughter, *Olivia*, and her boyfriend, *Kevin,* were waiting to take us to Mequon. Kevin (an African American) and Olivia had been dating for several months and their relationship had blossomed into a serious romance. The ride from Mitchell Field to Mequon was pleasant and full of casual banter.

It took a few days to reacquaint ourselves with life in Wisconsin, especially with the COVID epidemic now in full swing. Among the changes that were now in place, restaurants, public places, and apartment buildings had established 'COVID rules', and the building where my apartment was located, The Newport, was no exception. Their rules included the caveat that receptionists, residents, and other people entering the building, were required to wear a mask that covered their nose and mouth.

A few weeks after our return, with those rules in mind, I drove from Mequon to Milwaukee to retrieve some belongings from my apartment. As I entered the lobby of The Newport, I noticed that the receptionist, a young black woman, was wearing her mask on her chin, perched well below her nose and mouth. I said to her in a loud voice, "That mask belongs over your nose and your mouth, not on your chin!".

She did not comply with that request, and instead she angrily responded, "I'll wear it any way I want to!" One word led to another and after a minute she screamed the N word at me, "You n*****, you n*****, you n*****!". Her tirade was soon followed by other unprintable curse words.

Dismayed and almost speechless by that unexpected exchange and I strode past her into the hallway leading to my apartment. A few minutes later, after having retrieved the items I had come for, I exited my apartment and passed through the lobby to get to my car. Neither she nor I spoke another word, but it was obvious that her mouth and nose were still uncovered by her mask. I never learned her name and I did not report the incident to Newport management. Too shocked, I guess.

I cannot recall ever saying the N word to anyone, nor had I ever witnessed a black person saying that word in any context to anyone else. But I knew from my general experience and knowledge that black people commonly used the N word among themselves, mostly in a social context, and usually in a less vehement tone.

Later that day, still unnerved by what had happened I returned home to Libby and told her about it. She seemed to be almost as upset as I had been. After a few minutes, the matter dropped from our conversation as we turned to other subjects, and by the evening the event had faded to the back of my mind.

The next day Libby and I, Olivia and Kevin, and her parents, Kim and Richard, went for dinner at The Wisconsin Club. Kevin and Olivia sat at a nearby table, well within earshot. The dinner began with a glass of wine. Shortly afterward, Libby turned and asked me to tell them about the event at The Newport.

I was well aware that Kevin and Olivia were nearby, and I began telling the story. Shortly after reaching the part where I repeated the N word three times in the same loud voice that the Newport receptionist had used, Olivia stood up, took Kevin by the hand and exited from the dining room without saying a word.

Libby was surprised at what had transpired, and embarrassed that she had asked me to tell that story. The remainder of our dinner was eaten in silence, and we left the club shortly after finishing our food.

The next day I received a text message from Olivia who berated me for having spoken the N word in Kevin's presence. I realized that it had been insensitive to disregard Kevin's presence without at least qualifying what I was about to say. I immediately apologized in a return text to both of them. Olivia was unforgiving and replied that they would no longer interact with me. I had no reply.

A few days after that episode I sensed that something had changed between Libby and me. I knew that she loved Olivia and was devoted to her. I'm certain that she blamed herself for suggesting that I tell the story, but still uncertain whether she had reached the threshold where she felt forced to choose between love for me and that for Olivia. Whether my reasoning was correct or not, I believe that this event initiated the decline in our relationship.

Disenchantment

In July 2020, Libby put her Florida home on the market, and by that October she had closed the sale. During that same period, still convinced that our arrangement was solid and enduring, I put my Newport apartment on the market. It made sense for me to monetize the value of a place that I rarely used. It also was a way of signaling to Libby that I was 'all-in' as far as our staying together was concerned. When I told her about my plans, she was pleased and supportive.

In February, I accepted an offer for the apartment with a closing date at the end of April. Since Libby had been supportive throughout the period of marketing and sale of my apartment, I was confident that our relationship would not change. I was wrong!

During the downsizing process, I disposed of nearly all my furniture and other material belongings, including the Marshall & Wendell baby grand piano that had been in my possession for more than 75 years. By the time I vacated my unit, there were very few large items that remained. On moving day, I brought with me two desk chairs, one of which was for Libby's use, plus several cartons containing clothing, framed pictures, paintings, photo albums, CDs, a laser printer, my personal files, dishware, crystalware, silverware, and my golf clubs.

At the end of July, after years of what I had long regarded as a loving and blissful situation, Libby's behavior changed. One morning during breakfast she turned to me and blurted out that she wanted to live by herself. I was taken aback by her aggressiveness. She also added the trope that she had no intention of becoming my caregiver.

Earlier that month she had been busy organizing a 'Temkin family reunion' that would take place in Tarrytown, New York in September. I was invited and had recently booked our flights while Libby took care of hotel reservations.

During the four years we were together I had attended many Temkin family gatherings, including a most enjoyable trip to Chile. I had become friendly with many clan members including Todd and his family, Kim and Richard Taylor, Olivia and Ben Taylor, *Larry Temkin*, *Terri Temkin*, and several other relatives and friends.

In the middle of August, Libby added a complication to what had by then become a stressful situation. She abruptly announced that she didn't want me to attend the September reunion. Her explanation for that seemed absurd, namely that she wanted to spend her time at the reunion with her family, and she did not want to be concerned with my welfare or entertainment. It was painful to be rejected on such specious grounds, but nevertheless, I acceded to her demand.

It was now clear that staying with her at Hidden Reserve was no longer a viable option. I stopped sleeping with her and instead spent my nights in one of the guest rooms. We hardly spoke. I stepped up my search for a new living arrangement, and after a few weeks, I decided on Newcastle Place, a senior living community in Mequon about three miles from Hidden Reserve, and on October 22nd I did so.

The Rest of the Story[22]

As the date for the Temkin reunion drew closer I was still puzzled by the recent sequence of events. Libby and I had been together for nearly five years. We had shared an intimate and loving relationship for nearly that entire period. For a while I clung to the hope that, somehow, we might find a way to patch things up.

----

[22] The subtitle channels the late radio broadcaster, *Paul Harvey*, who was famous for interjecting memorable phrases such as *'page two'* and *'now for the rest of the story'* into his narrations.

Todd and his family had planned to visit Libby in Mequon immediately following the reunion, and I was hoping to see him at the time of their visit. During the previous four years we had become friends, or so I thought. We had played golf together several times, I enjoyed meeting his friends, and learning about his spirituality and his plans for developing his ranch in Futaleufú, Patagonia.

As described above, a few weeks before we were scheduled to leave for the Temkin reunion Libby asked me to remain at home and I complied. Shortly after her return from that meeting, she added that she didn't want me to be at home when Todd and his family visited. That request was hurtful and demeaning, and I asked for an explanation. The following is the gist of her response.

Two years earlier, during a Todd Temkin family visit to Boca Grove from their home in Chile, I reportedly had had several 'confrontations' with Todd's wife, Pilar. Because of those purported events, Libby did not want new incidents to occur during their forthcoming visit to Mequon, and that was why she asked me to leave.

That was the first I had heard about 'confrontations with Pilar'. I argued that the accusations were unfounded, but these entreaties had no effect. Reluctantly, I booked a week's stay at The Four Points Hotel in Brown Deer. [23]

---

[23] It is worth interjecting here that I had been briefed by Libby about Pilar's sociopathic, narcissistic, and manipulative behavior that she herself had experienced. As told to me by her, Todd, her husband, was often the object of her anti-utopian antics. Despite their degrading nature, Todd always tried to patch things up, reportedly in the interest of keeping their family together. Having been forewarned about these behavioral aberrancies, I decided early on that my interactions with Pilar would always be respectful, appropriately responsive, and never 'confrontational. I kept my word.

In searching my memories of that visit to Boca Grove I recalled a single interaction that might have been regarded as a confrontation by Pilar. On that occasion, instead of our usual process of having dinner at a restaurant, I offered to make dinner for everyone that evening at home. Pilar stared at me silently, turned toward her children and without comment, she escorted them to their automobile and drove off. I immediately told Libby about this incident she shrugged it off. A few hours later Pilar returned and without saying a word, she escorted her children upstairs for the night. That was perplexing.

On the morning of their expected arrival in Milwaukee, I was packed and prepared to depart for my hotel, but rather than leave immediately I went to the kitchen to await their arrival. No sooner had I settled into a chair, Libby shouted angrily, demanding to know why I had not left yet. I tried to explain but she became more adamant and shouted that she did not want me to be there when they arrived. Totally defeated by her words, I exited and headed for the hotel.

Later that day, I received this message from her:

"Hi Michael, I am writing this to you because I felt absolutely awful when you left this morning. That whole scene was so painful for both of us, and I need to apologize and tell you my thoughts. There was no reason for you not to have been here when Todd and his family arrived. I was just thinking that I wanted to avoid any confrontation that might have occurred. They really don't have the full understanding of our relationship, (sometimes we don't either), and could have misinterpreted it, making it uncomfortable for all of us. I should have been able to see through that, and I didn't, so I'm truly sorry. It really isn't up to them to define us, anyhow."

"I know you were hurt, when you left, and I was also. This whole time has been very difficult, I only wanted us to live apart, not give up on each other. There's a big difference."

The following day I received an email message from Todd that exposed his role in this fiasco:

"As you know well, my wife has a very strong personality. Even though we had a fantastic time with you in Patagonia, I still recall vividly the very difficult 3 weeks we spent under the same roof in Boca Grove several years ago, as we awaited Pilar's green card to return to Chile. There were many awkward and painful moments during those 3 weeks between you and Pilar. (I am not adjudicating blame. I am simply stating objective fact.)"

"It was me who floated to Mom the idea that it might be better if you considered spending this week with your family or in a hotel, not because I don't care for you, but because I didn't want to relive the awkwardness of Boca."

It was now clear that Libby's assertions of 'confrontations' with Pilar had been 'second-hand' tales that Todd had transmitted to his mother. To put a finer point on this, he had *not* been present to witness the so-called painful moments.

I wrote to him again that I had no recollection of any confrontation with Pilar during their visit, and asked him to explain the oxymoron, *'objective facts'*. After two days passed without a response, I wrote again. There was no reply.

Two days after receiving Todd's letter, Libby sent me another message under the subject line, "Some other thoughts", which are excerpted below:

"... Michael, I have had intense conversations with my grandchildren and everyone else concerned about last Friday morning. It was wrong and I want them to know that I'll talk to you when I get back Monday."

Although I appreciated her attempt to 'right the wrong', there was no reason to believe that she would attribute any blame to Pilar or Todd, or that she understood the baseless nature of their assertions. I was certain that Libby would never dispute her beloved son's version of events.

One month later I departed from Hidden Reserve and

moved to Newcastle Place. I had been *Libb-erated*!

After spending my first days at Newcastle Place, I wrote another letter to Todd, who had by then, returned with his family to Chile [*Addendum*]. The intent was to leave no doubt that I was aware of his complicity in promulgating Pilar's version of events. I asked him to justify his behavior. I also was certain that my letter would inevitably find its way to Libby, and that would only worsen the situation. But at that point, I no longer cared.

A day later I received a reply from Todd. He offered no coherent explanation for his behavior, and he did acknowledge that the slanderous accusations had originated with Pilar. He excused her behavior once again with, *'she has a very strong personality.'* He also admitted that he had not witnessed *'observable facts.'* Not surprisingly, shortly after receiving his response, I received an email from Libby who, as anticipated, was angry and annoyed that I had involved her son in this matter.

Final Words

After more than a year at Newcastle Place, I still could not fully understand why Libby's attitude toward me had changed so abruptly and completely. That ignorance might have continued indefinitely had I not received a 'seasons greeting' from *Larry Temkin*, Libby's nephew, which read:

"Dear Michael, I know that you are no longer seeing my aunt. But I still want to wish you a happy birthday (coming up). I hope this note finds you well, and that you are enjoying a wonderful holiday season."

I met Larry Temkin and his wife, Meg, on a visit to their home in New Jersey. That meeting took place a few months after the affair with Libby had begun. Larry is a 'Distinguished Professor of Philosophy'(Emeritus) at Rutgers University and a highly regarded authority in his field. His interests and expertise intersected with mine, and during a three-year period we

124

engaged in several illuminating discussions.

Larry's cordial message to me deserved a reply. In my response, I included a summary of the events that I believed had undermined our relationship. The next day I received his reply: "Dear Michael, I had heard about the breakup, and was sorry to hear about it. I know that my aunt greatly enjoyed your company for most of the time you were together. My aunt is a wonderful woman. And I love her dearly. But I was not surprised that she ended up breaking up with you. As you know, she had a hard time dealing with the decline of Sher, and she basically vowed she would never go through that again. I suspect that Todd's comments about how Pilar perceived you were more the proximate cause of the breakup, but not the ultimate cause. My own sense is that Aunt Libbie feared having to take care of you as you aged, and that was too much for her to deal with in the anticipation. This is not something you really had any control over. If I'm right, it just reflected Aunt Lib's deep fear of having to be the caregiver of an aging partner again. She just wasn't up to facing that. Warmly yours, Larry."

That letter was the wakeup call that I needed. After reading his message I could no longer minimize what should have been obvious long ago, namely that the basis for dissolution of our relationship was Libby's fear of becoming a caregiver again. The way that other more peripheral events that unfolded, provided her with a convenient exit ramp, and the complete collapse of our relationship.

Writing about times spent with the Temkin tribe has provided a pathway to closure. Despite everything that has happened, I am still unalterably bound to fond thoughts of Libby Temkin. I am grateful to her for having been the instrument of my recovery from grieving over Shirley's death, as well as for bringing so much happiness into my life for so many years. I wish her well.

Michael Mosesson

ADDENDUM
Letter to Todd Temkin, November 10, 2021

"I am writing to you today because I want to set the record straight about your and Pilar's false accusations about my behavior toward her three years ago. As you are aware, you sent me a letter on September 14, 2021, in which you detailed the basis for Libby's inexplicable demand that I cancel my planned trip to the Temkin Reunion and subsequently to vacate her home during the period you and your family were staying with her. Libby's requests were shocking, they were hurtful, and more importantly, they were incomprehensible. I could not understand why she would make such unqualified demands, but your letter at least clarified the 'why' and the 'who' of it. After receiving that letter I responded to you twice at Libby's email address. I received no response to either of the notes—it is not clear whether you even read them. What is clear is you did not respond.

Considerable time has passed since those letters were written, and that period included your brief return visit last month. I wanted to meet with you in person during your visit but there was insufficient time to arrange that meeting. Accordingly, I am writing this letter to clarify, explain, and expand my views.

Two months have passed since the September Temkin reunion and your family's visit to Mequon. Since then I have moved from Hidden Reserve to Newcastle Place, have nearly severed my relationship with Libby, and by extension, with everyone else in the Temkin family. From my standpoint, that is a regrettable and seemingly irreversible outcome.

I've had time to think about each event leading to this present situation. By writing, I hope to make you fully aware of the damage you caused on behalf of Pilar and her imagined complaints. By acceding to her admonitions, you evidently became convinced that there was substance to her accusations, in particular that she and I had had 'confrontations' during your 'Green Card' visit to Boca Grove. I searched my memory carefully and could not recall even one event that could be characterized as a 'confrontation' with her, let alone the 'awkward and painful moments' you averred in your letter. For the record and for your information, I unequivocally deny any and all accusations or behavioral aberrations that you or she raised, and those that Libby dutifully transmitted based upon your discussions with her.

Michael"

ACKNOWLEDGEMENTS

I am grateful to *Seth Banks* for reviewing this manuscript and for providing constructive comments and suggestions, as well as an endorsement. I also acknowledge *Kathy Kovacic* for her contributions to the cover design, and *lisa roma* who edited the text manuscript, fine-tuned the formatting and layout of this book.

I also wish to honor the memory of my longtime colleague and friend *John S. Finlayson*, a linguist, scholar, and scientist who helped me hone my writing abilities, who graciously and critically reviewed many of my published manuscripts, and who contributed a chapter to volume one of *Fibrinogen Memoirs*.

ABOUT THE AUTHOR AND THE TRILOGY

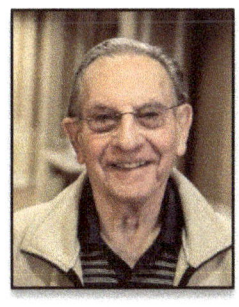 Michael Mosesson grew up in Brooklyn, New York. He earned his medical degree at SUNY Downstate Medical Center, and afterward spent more than fifty years as a hospital/medical school-based physician, teacher, and scientist. His clinical activities included internal medicine and hematology, with special attention to bleeding and thrombotic disorders, and fibrinolytic therapy. Mosesson's bench and clinical research activities focused mainly on fibrinogen, fibrin, fibrinolysis, thrombosis, and bleeding.

After finally ending his research activities at the *Blood Research Institute* of The Blood Center of Wisconsin, he turned to writing *Fibrinogen Memoirs* to slake his thirst for clarity and exposition.

Volume 1 is a compendium that ranges from his childhood to the present, covers personal experiences and recollections (including vivid descriptions from his career as a pilot), presentations of a variety of scientific subjects, historical events and accomplishments, plus recollections involving noteworthy investigators, Nobel laureates, cherished colleagues, friends, and family. The final chapter, written by John Finlayson, is concerned with events and personnel involved in the transition of the Laboratory of Blood and Blood Products at NIH to become a subsidiary of the Food and Drug Administration.

Fibrinogen Memoirs 2 provides an insightful and authoritative analysis of the controversy about the *structure of cross-linked fibrin clots*. The narrative is garnished with caricatures and bio-sketches of participants in the controversy.

The stories in *Fibrinogen Memoirs 3* are linked to one life-changing event in the author's medical career, as described in chapter one.

NAMES CITED (by chapter)

Abdoo, Bob (3)
Alkjaersig, Norma (8)
Amrani, David (3)
Anderson, Charles (8)
Anfinsen, Christian (2)
Ariens, Robert (5)
Aspect, Alain (2)
Barnard, Christian (3)
Bishop, Paul (5)
Butler, Samuel (4)
Castle, William (1)
Cayce, Edwin (9)
Christensen, Carl (3)
Church, Gil (7)
Clark, Barney (3)
Clauser, John (2)
Collins, Jean (9)
Cooley, Denton (3)
Crawford, Cindy (3)
Crick, Francis (2)
Cruise, Tom (6)
Cudahy, Michael (3)
Curley, James (1)
Damadian, Raymond (2)
Davidson, Charles (1)
Dembrow, Beth (9)
Dembrow, Judith (9)
Dennis, Clarence (1, 8)
DeVries, William (3)
DiCera, E (4)
Diedrich, Alicia (7)
Dock, William (1)

Doolittle, Russ (4, 5)
Duckler, Selma (nee: Lindenberg) (10)
Eckmann, Christian (9)
Eckmann, Sebastian Benjamin Anthony (9)
Eichna, Ludwig (2)
Farrell, David (4)
Finlayson, John S (1, 3)
Flemma, Robert J (3)
Fletcher, Tony (8)
Franklin, Rosalind (2)
Furchgott, Robert (2)
Galanis, John (3)
Gao, Hua (3)
Gelman, Andrew (4)
Graham, Billy (2)
Grunau, Gary (3)
Harvey, Paul (10)
Hatley, John (8)
Hudy, Bob (7)
Hudy, Lynn (7)
Jacob, Harry (1)
Kambol, Bill (9)
Kambol, Emma Grace (9)
Kambol, Luca (9)
Lauterbur, Paul (2)
Lee, T.D. (2)
Lelkes, Peter (3)
Maki, Jim (7, 8)
Mansfield, Peter (2)
Maroney, Jim (6)
Maroney, Susan (6)
Mast, Alan (6)
McDowell, Shirley Ann (8)

McNair, Charlie (3)
Medved, Leonid (5)
Ménaché, Doris (9)
Merigan, Thomas (1)
Michelangelo (2)
Minkoff, Larry (2)
Minot, George (1)
Moaddel, Maia (4)
Mosesson, Aimee Francine (8)
Mosesson, Amber (nee: Yost) (9)
Mosesson, Arden (9)
Mosesson, Benjamin (9)
Mosesson, Esther (8,9)
Mosesson, Harper (9)
Mosesson, Marni Helene (8)
Mosesson, Matthew Norman (8, 9)
Mosesson, Shirley Ann (McDowell) (10)
Murphy, William (1)
Nackman, Les (8)
Nikolaychik, Victor (3)
Nirenberg, Marshall (2)
Partleton, Jim (7)
Pierce, William (3)
Prusiner, Stanley (2)
Richards, Arnie (nee: Gurodowski) (10)
Rieselbach, Richard (3)
Rocco, Mattia (3,5)
Schenker, Victor (1)
Schmidt, Donald H (3)
Schmidt, Mary Kay (3)
Sender, Adrienne (10)
Sender, Neville (10)
Shapiro, Sandor (Sandy) (1)

Shattil, Sandy (Sanford) (4)
Sherry, Sol (8)
Siebenlist, Kevin (4)
Smith, Luke (3)
Stone, Dr. (9)
Taylor, Ben (10)
Taylor, Kim Temkin (10)
Taylor, Olivia (10)
Taylor, Richard (10)
Temkin, Larry (8,10)
Temkin, Libby (8,10)
Temkin, Meg (10)
Temkin, Pilar (10)
Temkin, Robyn (10)
Temkin, Sher (10)
Temkin, Terrie (10)
Temkin, Todd (10)
Uecker, Bob (3)
Watson, James (2)
Weisel, John (5)
Whipple, George (1)
Wilkins, Maurice (2)
Wolf, Marilynn (8)
Wu, Shiung Chien (2)
Yang, Chen Ming (2)
Zellinger, Anton (2)

www.ingramcontent.com/pod-product-compliance
Lightning Source LLC
Chambersburg PA
CBHW051207120626
46547CB00013B/1242